MEDICAL RADIOLOGY
Radiation Oncology

Editors:
L. W. Brady, Philadelphia
H.-P. Heilmann, Hamburg
M. Molls, Munich
C. Nieder, Bodø

P. Rubin · L. S. Constine
L. B. Marks · P. Okunieff (Eds.)

CURED I · LENT
Late Effects of Cancer Treatment on Normal Tissues

With Contributions by

M. J. Adams · M. S. Anscher · N. M. Aziz · S. Bhatia · C. Bole · D. J. Brenner
J. M. Brown · E. P. Cohen · C. N. Coleman · L. S. Constine · L. F. Fajardo L-G
C. Figuero-Moseley · M. Fordis · O. Gayou · E. J. Hall · D. E. Hallahan · R. P. Hill
M. Hofman · M. Horowitz · M. M. Hudson · M. J. Joines · M. E. Kaufman
M. A. Kahn · Z. Kocak · W. Landier · A. R. Langan · S. E. Lipshultz · L. B. Marks
A. T. Meadows · M. Miften · G. R. Morrow · J. E. Moulder · K. M. Mustian
K. C. Oefinger · P. Okunieff · D. S. Parda · D. Poplack · R. G. Prosnitz · J. A. Roscoe
P. Rubin · L. Shankar · C. Sklar · D. C. Sullivan · J. Van Dyk · Z. Vuyaskovic
C. D. Willey · I. W. T. Yeung

Foreword by
L. W. Brady, H.-P. Heilmann, M. Molls, and C. Nieder

With 54 Figures in 68 Separate Illustrations, 30 in Color and 26 Tables

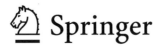

Philip Rubin, MD
Professor Emeritus
Chair Emeritus
Department of Radiation Oncology
University of Rochester
School of Medicine and Dentistry
601 Elmwood Avenue, Box 647
Rochester, NY 14642
USA

Louis S. Constine, MD
Professor of Radiation Oncology and Pediatrics
Vice Chair, Department of Radiation Oncology
Departments of Radiation Oncology and Pediatrics
University of Rochester
School of Medicine and Dentistry
601 Elmwood Avenue, Box 647
Rochester, NY 14642
USA

Lawrence B. Marks, MD
Professor
Department of Radiation Oncology
Duke University Medical Center
P.O. Box 3085
Durham, NC 27710
USA

Paul Okunieff, MD
Philip Rubin Professor of Radiation Oncology
Chair, Department of Radiation Oncology
University of Rochester
School of Medicine and Dentistry
601 Elmwood Avenue, Box 647
Rochester, NY 14642
USA

Medical Radiology · Diagnostic Imaging and Radiation Oncology
Series Editors:
A. L. Baert · L. W. Brady · H.-P. Heilmann · M. Knauth · M. Molls · C. Nieder · K. Sartor

Continuation of Handbuch der medizinischen Radiologie
Encyclopedia of Medical Radiology

ISBN 978-3-642-08032-6   e-ISBN 978-3-540-49070-8

This work is subject to copyright. All rights are reserved, whether the whole or part of the material is concerned, specifically the rights of translation, reprinting, reuse of illustrations, recitations, broadcasting, reproduction on microfilm or in any other way, and storage in data banks. Duplication of this publication or parts thereof is permitted only under the provisions of the German Copyright Law of September 9, 1965, in its current version, and permission for use must always be obtained from Springer-Verlag. Violations are liable for prosecution under the German Copyright Law.

Springer is part of Springer Science+Business Media

http//www.springer.com

© Springer-Verlag Berlin Heidelberg 2010

The use of general descriptive names, trademarks, etc. in this publication does not imply, even in the absence of a specific statement, that such names are exempt from the relevant protective laws and regulations and therefore free for general use.

Product liability: The publishers cannot guarantee the accuracy of any information about dosage and application contained in this book. In every case the user must check such information by consulting the relevant literature.

Medical Editor: Dr. Ute Heilmann, Heidelberg
Desk Editor: Ursula N. Davis, Heidelberg
Production Editor: Kurt Teichmann, Mauer
Cover-Design and Typesetting: Verlagsservice Teichmann, Mauer

Printed on acid-free paper – 21/3180xq – 5 4 3 2 1 0

Dedications

Dedication to Robert Kallman
LENT V Scientific Meeting

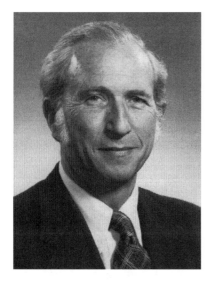

Fig. 1. Robert Kallman, PhD

Bob was an inspiration to all of us and to many others in approaching all activities with a gusto and enthusiasm that was quite extraordinary. Those who knew Bob also remember his enthusiasm for the outdoors, in particular skiing, kayaking, and fishing. Those who skied with him will not easily forget the image of Bob, apparently barely in control as he sped down the slopes arms flailing, but rarely wiping out. His will to live as full a life as possible was exemplified by a trip to the Radiation Research Society meeting in Reno, even though he was wheeling an oxygen bottle with him. And he made all the tailgate parties at Stanford football games in his final year under the same circumstances.

Bob's research interests were in tumor hypoxia and in the combination of chemotherapeutic drugs and radiation. He identified and characterized, with his colleague, Luke van Putten of the Netherlands, the phenomenon of reoxygenation of tumors following irradiation. He published a hundred or so research articles and edited a very influential book on rodent tumor models in experimental cancer therapy (Rodent tumor models in experimental cancer therapy. Pergamon Press, New York, 1987). This is still the "bible" for people measuring tumor response to therapy today. He was an active member of the Radiation Research Society, and served as its 25th president from 1976–1977. Bob stepped down from his major administrative roles in 1984, devoted more time to his research, and retired in 1992.

One of Bob's most lasting contributions – certainly to Stanford and to the many graduates of the program – was his founding, in 1978, of Stanford's Cancer Biology Program, of which he served as its first Director for 6 years. Founding this program was no small feat. The opposition within the University to having a graduate program based on a disease was enormous and it is unquestionably a tribute to Bob's persistence and powers of persuasion that it ever got off the ground. The grant he received from the National Cancer Institute to fund the program is currently in its 25th uninterrupted year and there are currently some 50 graduate students and a half-dozen postdocs currently in the program. I got my start in radiobiology – particularly my interest in tumor hypoxia – under Bob's tutelage, as a postdoctoral fellow when I first came to Stanford. Ironically, when he died on August 8, 2003, after a lengthy battle with lung disease, it was hypoxia and his inability to reoxygenate that let to his demise.

Born May 21, 1922, in Brooklyn, NY, Bob grew up in Woodmere, Long Island, NY, and attended Hofstra College, receiving his A.B. in 1943. He served as a medic in the US Army in Europe during World War II. He attended graduate school at New

York University, receiving a PhD in biology in 1952. With his first wife, Frances "Pat" Green, he moved to the west coast in 1952 to take up a position at the Radiological Laboratory at the University of California at San Francisco. Bob is survived by his second wife Ingrid, and his children, Tim Kallman of Cabin John, MD, Robin Kallman of San Francisco, and Lars Kallman of Stanford; two grandchildren, Maria and Benji Kallman; his sister, Nancy Rudolph of New York City; his brother, Raymond Kallman of Taos, NM; and numerous nieces and nephews.

Bob was amongst the founding faculty members of the new Palo Alto Medical School campus in 1956 when he was recruited by Henry Kaplan to create a Division of Radiation Biology. It is important to note that both Henry and Bob together moved the clinical discipline of radiation oncology, largely empirical, onto a scientific basis by pioneering translational research at Stanford and NIH. That is, by modeling in the laboratory, using small animals, they tested novel forms of treatment(s) prior to their introduction to patients via randomized clinical trials. The standard for excellence in radiation oncology research was set by Bob Kallman whose fervor recruited a number of creative PhD faculty members such as Kendric Smith, George Hahn, and myself. In addition, virtually all of the newly recruited clinical faculty were inspired to have active research projects and included Mal Begshaw, Zvi Fuks, and Norman Coleman, to mention a few notable investigators. Bob Kallman was continually funded by NIH grants throughout his career, as was his faculty. By being active in NIH peer review visits, his template for excellence in oncologic radiation research became a national reality.

It is often said that with due modesty my career began by standing on the shoulder of a giant. Bob, in real life, was a giant of a man and the metaphor could be applied not only figuratively but literally in all of his life's venues and appetites. His passion for travel, his exquisite recall of precise details, his palette for gourmet food and vintage wines were raconteured with delight. His quest for the scientific truth, finding a defining insight at the bench, was matched by his zeal for finding fresh powder on mountain trails. His legacy is his lasting imprimatur on the minds of colleagues on all of the world's continents and on the hearts of faculty, fellows, residents, and graduate students, many of whom have lead newly formed Divisions of Radiation Biology and/or chaired Departments of Radiation Oncology. But most of all he will be remembered for his esprit de coeur, that energetic spirit he infused with such generosity for those who were his friends and brethren.

J. MARTIN BROWN

Eric J. Hall:
The Radiobiologist's Radiobiologist

The Eric Hall story started a few years ago in Abertillery, in South Wales, where a promising rugby career (Fig. 1) was forsaken for the bright lights of London, and from there to the hallowed halls of Oxford University. In Oxford, Eric met a pivotal figure in his career, Frank Ellis, and was soon drawn into the world of radiotherapy.

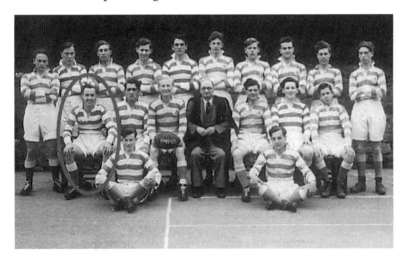

Fig. 1. The promising rugby player

Hall's first contributions were in medical physics, designing compensators for variations in tissue thickness [1], very much in the Frank Ellis spirit of treating every patient as an individual challenge. But it was not long before he was drawn to the radiobiological underpinnings of radiotherapy, and the three themes that have dominated his career so far soon became apparent.

The first Hall theme, first appearing in 1961 [2], is RBE, the relative biological effect of one radiation compared to another – assayed with bean roots and, as mammalian cells became available for radiobiological study, with rodent and human cells. Interestingly, while Hall became known worldwide for characterizing RBEs of more esoteric radiations, such as neutrons [3] and charged particles [4], his first RBE paper [2] was on the RBE of X-rays compared to gamma rays. His 1961 conclusion, that keV X-rays and MeV gamma rays have significantly different RBEs, is as pertinent today as it was then. The ICRP, who worry interminably about the RBEs of neutrons and charged particles, but much less about different energy photons [5], would do well to read this classic [2], and the follow-up papers [6].

The second Hall theme is the effect of dose rate and fractionation, initially stemming from a collaboration with Joel Bedford [7, 8], when Hall first visited the US as a Fulbright scholar. The Bedford/Hall dose-rate schematic (Fig. 2) must be the most reproduced figure in the history of radiobiology. Hall has revisited this dose rate theme repeatedly, making critical contributions to many of the new alternate fractionation modalities, such as high dose rate brachytherapy, pulsed dose rate, and hypofractionation.

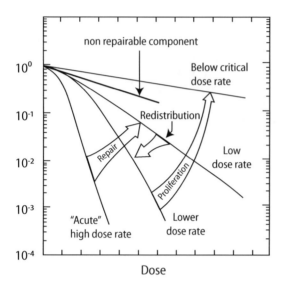

Fig. 2. The radiobiology of dose rate, Bedford and Hall style

The third Hall theme is hypoxia [9]. Over the years, probably no other topic has vexed radiobiologists more. Hypoxia affects radiosensitivity, of this there is no doubt, but the overarching theme of Hall's research soon became apparent when, in 1967, he asked whether the oxygen effect is "pertinent or irrelevant to clinical radiotherapy?" [10]. The answer has remained tantalizingly elusive, but it's a rare paper on clinical hypoxia that does not quote Hall.

By 1967, Hall had met Harald Rossi and moved to Columbia University in New York City (Fig. 3). Their collaboration set the tone for how radiobiology was approached for the next several decades, worldwide, with the physics and chemistry of energy deposition integrally linked with radiobiology [11]. In that context, their collaboration was extraordinarily fruitful, and laid the foundations for the way in which a generation of radiation researchers went about their business. In the last decade, as the tools of the genomic revolution have become available, this symbiotic relationship between the physical and the biological sciences has become less common. Not, it seems, for good scientific reasons, but more because molecular biologists are simply not trained in the physical sciences. The radiation field is suffering significantly because of this schism, and might do well to reconsider the Rossi-Hall academic model.

But back to one of Hall's themes that is very much alive and well, and that is training young clinicians. Radiobiology for the Radiologist is the unchallenged text book in the field, from the first edition in 1973 up to the sixth edition in 2005. It's not just for clinicians: if anyone wants to get up to speed fast about some particular area of radiobiology, a clear, concise summary is sure to be found in the book. The theme of teaching young clinicians was never clearer than at ASTRO, where Hall taught his two part course on "Radiation and Cancer Biology" to generations of clinicians.

To summarize this mid-term report on the scientific career of Eric Hall so far: First, early, he spotted and persisted with the three great themes of radiobiology, RBE, dose rate, and hypoxia. Second, he has never lost sight of why these are important topics – the clinic. Third, he has communicated these themes with erudition and passion to generations of clinicians and basic scientists. Not bad, so far….

DAVID J. BRENNER

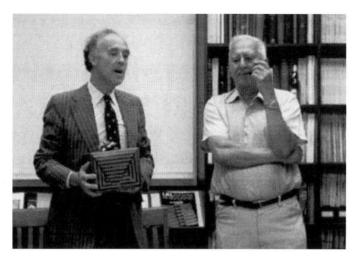

Fig. 3. Eric Hall and Harald Rossi

REFERENCES

1. Ellis F, Hall EJ, Oliver R (1959) A compensator for variations in tissue thickness for high energy beams. Br J Radiol 32:421–422
2. Hall EJ (1961) The relative biological efficiency of X-rays generated at 220 kVp and gamma radiation from a cobalt 60 therapy unit. Br J Radiol 34:313–317
3. Hall EJ (1969) Radiobiological measurements with 14 MeV neutrons. Br J Radiol 42:805–813
4. Hall EJ (1973) Radiobiology of heavy particle radiation therapy: cellular studies. Radiology 108:119–129
5. ICRP (1991) Recommendations of the International Commission on Radiological Protection: Publication 60. Pergamon, Oxford
6. Borek C, Hall EJ, Zaider M (1983) X-rays may be twice as potent as gamma rays for malignant transformation at low doses. Nature 301:156–158
7. Hall EJ, Bedford JS (1964) Dose rate: its effect on the survival of HeLa cells irradiated with gamma rays. Radiat Res 22:305–315
8. Hall EJ, Bedford JS (1964) A Comparison of the effects of acute and protracted gamma-radiation on the growth of seedlings of Vicia Faba. I. Experimental observations. Int J Radiat Biol Relat Stud Phys Chem Med 8:467–474
9. Hall EJ, Cavanagh J (1967) The oxygen effect for acute and protracted radiation exposures measured with seedlings of Vicia Faba. Br J Radiol 40:128–133
10. Hall EJ (1967) The oxygen effect: pertinent or irrelevant to clinical radiotherapy? Brit J Radiol 40:874–875
11. Hall EJ, Kellerer AM, Rossi HH, Lam YM (1978) The relative biological effectiveness of 160 MeV protons – II. Biological data and their interpretation in terms of microdosimetry. Int J Radiat Oncol Biol Phys 4:1009–1013

Dedication to Richard L. Levy and Timothy E. Guertin

Tracing the Trajectory of Cancer Curability
The Ascent of the Linac as the Icon for Cancer Cure

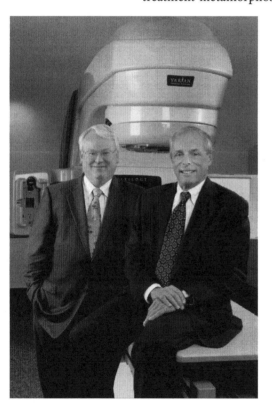

Fig. 1. Richard L. Levy, CEO, and Timothy E. Guertin, President, with Linac of Varian Medical Systems

Tracing the trajectory of cancer curability demonstrates how the source for radiation treatment metamorphosed from a simple one-dimensional stationary object, the cathode X-ray tube – virtually unchanged at mid-century in the 1950s – into a multidimensional dynamic megavoltage, variable energy, dual photon and electron beam, highly computerized, multileaf collimation radiation-delivery system, capable of 360° rotation, extremely high dose rates, pulsatile gated in coordination with a moving target, the malignancy to be eradicated. The curability of cancer was an abstraction, a problem to be solved in the 1950s when orthovoltage, kilovoltage machines were utilized by all radiologists for both diagnosis and treatment of neoplastic diseases. The curability of cancer and the emergence of Radiation Oncology as a distinct medical specialty, based on the radiologic sciences of physics and biology, are in a large measure due to the development and dissemination of the linear accelerator over five continents in five decades. The "Varian Linacs" are the metaphor for radiation cancer curability as we enter into the new millennium. It is for making the abstract idea of "cancer cure" a reality, with normal tissue and organ preservation, while extending the survival of millions of afflicted patients, that we honor Richard L. Levy by dedicating this issue to him on his retirement as President and CEO of Varian Medical System, Inc., and to his constant deputy and successor, Timothy E. Guertin, the new President (Fig. 1).

The transformation of the ordinary to that dimension of the extraordinary began after WWII with the Varian brothers, who decided to build a klystron 1000 times more powerful than any built during wartime. This lead to the "traveling wave guide" by which radar-like waves are pulsed into a microwave power source (the klystron); electrons are then emitted from a hot cathode and ride the radar like waves, much like a surfer riding an ocean wave curl. As electrons increasingly gain energy from traveling the waves, they exit at high velocity. This seminal concept was transformed into a compact size configuration as an elongated tubular machine that could oscillate through a 360° angle from vertical to horizontal. With Henry Kaplan's vision of developing the ideal megavoltage clinical accelerator, Gintzon and Hansen, Professors of physics, were inspired and together synergized clinical dreams into a real world.

Their seminal technologic stream resulted in the radiation therapy Linac. It was truly an apocryphal moment and a real advent of translational research. Their abstract concept and design we now know proved to be the most advanced and optimal radiation delivery device to be applied medically for the cure of cancer in the twentieth century (Fig. 2).

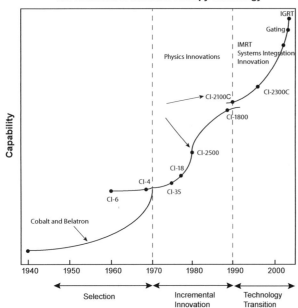

Fig. 2. Tracing the trajectory of the incremental seminal technologic stream provided by physicians and physicists allowed the Linac to be the most advanced and optimal radiation delivery device in the 20th century.

Following their initiative, the Radiation Medical Division at Varian was formed in the 1960s. Due to a fortuitous concatenation of contiguous circumstances, Richard Levy, a young physicist, became the Director and Coordinator in the creative actualizing of the design of the Linac. His remarkable vision and tenacious pragmatism made the Linac the "enabling technology" for the emergence of Radiation Oncology as a distinct medical specialty. His sharp sense of economics and investment is reflected in the incremental gains in earnings over five decades. Rivaling Alan Greenspan's insights, Richard Levy's rise to president and CEO of Varian is a reflection of his managerial astuteness that in large measures led to Varian's commercial success.

The major innovations that resulted in a desirable technology trajectory are shown in Fig. 3. It was the traveling wave-guide that allowed for Linac design that gave Varian the leading edge commercially and resulted in their dominant position as the world's premier manufacturer. To understand the impact of these Linacs clinically we need to appreciate how these creative steps in physics provided new dimensions for the radiation oncologists to attack a variety of cancers from different directions and angles. The metamorphosis of the cathode X-ray tube into the modern linear accelerator transformed our discipline forever. The impetus for the separation of diagnosis and treatment into distinct specialties each with their own Boards, Societies, Journal, Sciences and NIH Grant Support was due to the separation of radiation instruments utilized by each discipline.

It required a decade for Varian to move into an assembly line production in the 1970s, but it wasn't until the 1980s when the supply reached the demand, production became profitable and the medical division of Varian, Inc., was the corporation's dominant activity and led to Richard Levy's promotion to President and CEO. The development of this linear accelerator technology has indirectly diminished the need for disposing of large quantities of radioactive waste material. By contrast, depreciated linear accelerators can be rehabilitated and indeed are given a second life in developing nations. Fortunately, within a matter of two decades (the 1980s and 1990s) the telecobalt units were phased out (Fig. 3).

As Radiation Oncology became more effective cancer became more curable with available multidisciplinary approaches. The NCI goal of curing 50% of all malignancies has been achieved as we enter this new millennium. The most dramatic illustration is in controlling childhood malignancies where advances in surgery, then radiation and chemotherapy lead to a dramatic reversal from inevitable cancer death to predictable cancer survival. The trajectory of pediatric tumor curability curve from 0% to 20% in 1950 for a variety of neoplasms rose to > 50%–90%. Equally important is the minimalization of adverse effects in long-term cancer survivors by synergistically combining modalities.

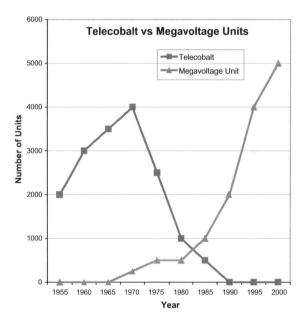

Fig. 3. Tracing the trajectory of the linear accelerator resulted in phasing out Telecobalt units over two decades.

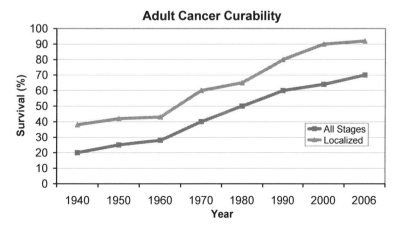

Fig. 4. Tracing the trajectory of adult cancer curability as 5-year survival rates (%) over five decades based on NCI SEER data

In adults, the gains in long-term survival have lead to halving cancer mortality by the year 2000. An analysis of US Bureau of Consensus and the NCI SEER data shows a significant improvement in 5-year survival rates by decade from 39% in the 1960s to 48% in the 1970s to 50% in the 1980s to 60% in the 1990s (Fig. 4). The gain in survival has occurred at 15–20 sites, most of which have reached significant levels. Too often the incremental improvement in an effective treatment as in radiation instrumentation is unheralded or not considered newsworthy. The sensationalizing of the latest exciting new finding in the laboratory is pronounced in news and video media as the proverbial answer to the management of the complexities of all cancers. The drug de jour, the designer molecule, the magical herbs of alternative medicine are touted highly but most, unfortunately, do not fulfill their promises in the grist of NCI oncologic clinical trials, which are the crucibles.

Conclusion

If the past is the prologue to the future, dynamic and innovative radiation treatment planning and delivery systems will be continually improving. Rather than radiation as a modality disappearing because of advances in chemotherapy, biologic response modifiers, immunomodulators and gene therapy, we have learned to be more effective by using radiation in combination with new and other modalities. The multidisciplinary approach to oncology has been established with cooperation and coordination rather than competition. The future promises that the Varian technologic trajectory is still ascending and on the rise….as is cancer curability.

Philip Rubin

Foreword

The rapid advances in radiation oncology, radiation biology, and radiation therapy physics have led to an accumulation of information on the interactions of radiation with other therapeutic modalities, such as the wide array of chemotherapeutic agents being employed in combination with radiation therapy, as well as the multiple biologic response modifiers that are being used in combination with radiation therapy. It is now recognized that they have a significant impact on normal tissue toxicities.

The radiation doses customarily deemed safe on the basis of past experience have now, when combined with other modalities, led to severe late effects in different vital organs. The previously defined radiation tolerance dosages remain as valuable guides, but their applicability has changed significantly. The emphasis is now placed on the volume of the organ irradiated, as well as the dose being used. New constructs relating global (whole organ) and focal (partial volume) injury as a function of the dose volume histogram emerge as a significant predictor of late effects on normal tissues. There are now mathematical models such as the model on standard dose, time–dose factors, and accumulated radiation effects that have been supplanted by linear-quadratic equations using the alpha/beta ratio and its clinical applicability to normal tissue complications.

This volume presents contemporary data relating to late effects on normal tissues. It is a composite of two symposia that were held at the University of Rochester. The papers presented at those two meeting are now compiled in this volume, making significantly important contributions to a better understanding of late effects on normal tissues.

The volume is dedicated to Dr. Robert Kallman, an outstanding investigator in radiation biology, as well as Dr. Eric Hall, an equally outstanding investigator in radiation oncology.

Arising from this conference is a better understanding of radiation in combination with other treatment modalities on late effects in normal tissues.

Philadelphia	Luther W. Brady
Hamburg	Hans-Peter Heilmann
Munich	Michael Molls
Bodø	Carsten Nieder

Introduction

Radiation Oncology Continuum: Cured Cancer Survivorship Research and Education (How our ugly duckling can become a beautiful swan!)

The search for the most favorable therapeutic ratio has been the "holy grail" quest of modern radiation oncology – namely ablating cancer with conservation and preservation of normal tissues. Our awareness of radiation associated late effects in the past century became further heightened as new modalities were introduced, i.e., megavoltage beams, computerized dynamic multileaf collimation for 3D conformal therapy, and high LET particles such as protons and neutrons. Heightened normal tissue reactions appeared with the escalation of radiation doses, bypass fractionated and accelerated fractionation, and aggressive combinations of concurrent chemotherapy and radiation regimens that have ablated more and more cancers. Our "well" cancer survivor enjoying a high quality of life is our reward and legacy. It is to achieve this goal that we advocate a multidisciplinary approach to caring for the cancer survivor after treatment as we have for the cancer patient during treatment.

The original biopathologic paradigm viewing acute and late effects in normal tissues following radiation as a biocontinuum of response and repair [1] applies to other modalities often combined with irradiation in multimodal treatment, i.e., chemotherapy, biologics, and surgery. The expression of a persistent toxicity over time has been shown by laboratory experimentation to be caused by a variety of cellular, tissue, environmental, and host factors. The radiation induction of DNA/RNA damage leading to a perpetual cascade of cytokine and chemokines, inducing inflammatory and profibrotic events is well appreciated. Ultimately, the histohematic barrier in the tissue interstitium leads to microvascular compromise and parenchymal cell atrophy. With high doses above tolerance there is the rapid onset of an arteritis of small feeder vessels within an organ due to thrombosis. If arterial occlusion is rapid, infarction and necrosis of the parenchyma occurs in contrast to a slow occlusion that leads to parenchymal cell atrophy and replacement fibrosis.

Starting in the 1980s, the NCI has supported a number of consensus meetings to develop common toxicity criteria (CTC), with the first two versions of the scales concerned with acute effects. Simultaneously, the RTOG in conjunction with other national and international cooperative groups began developing a late effects grading system. An agreement between RTOG and EORTC resulted in simultaneous publications in dedicated issues to SOMA categories in 1992 [2]. An NCI CTEP meeting in 2002 integrated LENT-SOMA into CTC Adverse Effects V3.0 and its subsequent publication alerted the major oncologic disciplines to a newly created NCI Office of Cancer Survivorship [3]. The contents of this issue are the summation of the LENT V NCI sponsored meeting in May, 2004, and addresses a number of critical topics related to late effects.

This year, the Institute of Medicine and the National Research Council issued an important document entitled "From Cancer Patient to Cancer Survivor – Lost in Transition" [4]. Its premise is the need to set a high priority to provide long-term follow-up care to the cured patient. The new millennium heralded the NCI goal of curing more than 50% of all malignancies. To be more specific, 85% of children and 60% of adults will survive cancer long term because of the multidisciplinary approach which is the cornerstone to success. Our country has more than 10 million survivors, and we are adding approximately 1,000,000 new cancer survivors annually. It is within this context that the contributions of radiation oncology, after decades of technologic and scientific advances, have become evident and are now well recognized and known. The signal cancers chosen for fuller discussion have extremely high survival rates of greater than 90%, i.e., prostate cancer, breast cancer, and Hodgkin's disease, and represent diseases in which the contributions of radiation oncology have been seminal.

The radiation oncology continuum conceptually can be viewed as a paradigm shift with the ever improving survival rates of cancer patients indicative of the permanency of curing cancer. That is, the continuum of cancer control parallels the normal tissue biocontinuum postradiation. The localized early cancer patients that are predominantly cancers of the prostate, breast, colorectum, urinary bladder, cervix, uterus, laryngopharynx, and Hodgkin's disease according to the most recent SEER/ACS cancer statistics have more than 90%–95% 5-year survival [5]. The vast majority of 5-year survivors will become 10-, 15-, even 20-year survivors. Thus, there is an increasing need because of the growing population of cancer survivors to promote health, prevent secondary disease and second malignant tumors, and to ensure their social, psychological, and economic well being. The research areas addressed in this issue relate to etiopathogenesis, screening, and early detection by biomarkers and bioimaging during its latent phase. The biointerventions and biopreventions optimally timed will decrease the morbidity and improve the quality of life. The ugly duckling of untoward late effects of cancer treatment by thoughtful, well-designed guidelines will assist health care providers to morph the cancer survivor into a beautiful swan.

PHILIP RUBIN and LOUIS SANDERS CONSTINE, III

References

1. Rubin P, Casarett G (1998) Clinical pathology, vols. I and II. WB Saunders, Philadelphia
2. Anonymous (1995) Late effects of normal tissues consensus conference. Int J Rad Onc Biol Phy 31:1035-1367
3. Trotti A, Rubin P (eds) (2003) The adverse effects of cancer treatments: metrics, management, and investigations. Semin Radiat Oncol 13:175
4. Hewitt M, Greenfield S, Stovall E (eds) (2006) From cancer patient to cancer survivor – lost in transition. The National Academies Press, Washington, D.C.
5. Ries LAG, Eisner MP, Kosary CL et al. (eds) (2004) SEER Cancer Statistics Review, 1975–2002, National Cancer Institute, Bethesda, MD

Acknowledgement

The RTOG/NCI support and sponsorship of periodic scientific workshops related to the "Late Effects of Normal Tissues" (LENT) has been ongoing for decades. There have been numerous corporate sponsors, the most persistent and generous being Varian Medical Systems.

- LENT IV Conference (1995) was dedicated to George Casarett.
- LENT V Conference (2005) honored Robert Kallman and was coincident with his birthday.
- LENT VI Conference recognized the transition to Cancer Survivorship Research and Education and became CURED I. This scientific meeting honored and recognized Eric Hall, not only for his contributions to radiation biology and oncology, but for his successful battle with prostate cancer. A cancer survivor for a decade, his enthusiasm for life, sailing, and skiing remains undiminished.
- This printing of Late Effects of Cancer Treatment on Normal Tissues is dedicated to Richard Levy and Tim Guertin, past President and current President of Varian, respectively, on the occasion of Richard's retirement as President.

This textbook volume owes its timely publication to Luther Brady and Peter Heilman who expeditiously recommended us to Springer. Ursula Davis, the managing editor, has been instrumental in the final collation of papers. Last, but certainly not least, special thanks are owed to the most dedicated project coordinator and editorial assistant, Heike Kross, who completed this project initiated by Amy Huser and persevered to bring this project to completion.

Finally, and most importantly, the inspiration and support for the CURED I meeting reflect my personal involvement in the long-term care of two of my Hodgkin's disease survivors, Mayer Mitchell (Stage IV) and Salvatore Bonacci (Stage III). Treated with total nodal irradiation and chemotherapy 40 years ago, they are more than close friends -- they are family. They have generously supported the Cancer Survivorship Research and Education (CURED) concept and LENT meetings at the University of Rochester when there was no other source of funding. Both have enjoyed active business and family lives, but, ironically, as this volume goes to press, both are facing life-threatening late effects of cancer treatment, i.e., second malignant cancers and valvular and coronary artery disease. It is the ongoing commitment to their care that has been the seeding and planting of the CURED program. It is fitting on behalf of all the authors contributing to the book to acknowledge that what matters most is the biocontinuum of care and caring for our cancer survivors.

We wish to recognize support from the NCI Conference Grant 1 R13 CA107566-01 and a grant by the RTOG cooperative group.

Contents

1 Radiation (and Medical) Biosurveillance: Screening Survivors for Late Effects of Therapy Using the Children's Oncology Group Long-Term Follow-Up Guidelines
Melissa M. Hudson, Wendy Landier, Smita Bhatia, Kevin C. Oeffinger, Charles Sklar, Anna Meadows, Marc Horowitz, David Poplack, Michael Fordis, and Louis S. Constine 1

2 Medical Countermeasures to Radiation Injury: Science and Service in the Public Interest. A Tribute to Robert Kallman
C. Norman Coleman 11

3 Ionizing Radiation and the Endothelium. A Brief Review
Luis Felipe Fajardo L-G... 19

4 Inflammation and Cell Adhesion Molecules are Involved in Radiation-Induced Lung Injury
Christopher D. Willey and Dennis E. Hallahan 23

5 Volume Effects in Radiation Damage to Rat Lung
Richard P. Hill, Mohammed A. Khan, Aimee R. Langan, Ivan W.T. Yeung, and Jake Van Dyk 31

6 The Role of Imaging in the Study of Radiation-Induced Normal Tissue Injury
Zafer Kocak, Lalitha Shankar, Daniel C. Sullivan, and Lawrence B. Marks 37

7 Screening for Cardiovascular Disease in Survivors of Thoracic Radiation
M. Jacob Adams, Robert G. Prosnitz, Louis S. Constine, Lawrence B. Marks, and Steven E. Lipshultz 47

8 Hypoxia-Mediated Chronic Normal Tissue Injury: A New Paradigm and Potential Strategies for Intervention
Mitchell Steven Anscher and Zeljko Vujaskovic................... 61

9 Prevention and Treatment of Radiation Injuries: The Role of the Renin-Angiotensin System
Eric P. Cohen, Melissa M. Joines, and John E. Moulder 69

10 Second Malignancies as a Consequence of Radiation Therapy
Eric J. Hall and David J. Brenner................................... 77

11 Using Quality of Life Information to Rationally Incorporate
   Normal Tissue Effects into Treatment Plan Evaluation and Scoring
   MOYED MIFTEN, OLIVIER GAYOU, DAVID S. PARDA,
   ROBERT PROSNITZ, and LAWRENCE B. MARKS 83

12 Cancer-Related Fatigue as a Late Effect: Severity in Relation to
   Diagnosis, Therapy, and Related Symptoms
   GARY R. MORROW, JOSEPH A. ROSCOE, MARALYN E. KAUFMAN,
   CHRISTOPHER BOLE, COLMAR FIGUEROA-MOSELEY,
   MAARTEN HOFMAN, and KAREN M. MUSTIAN 91

13 Normal Tissue TNM Toxicity Taxonomy:
   Scoring the Adverse Effects of Cancer Treatment
   PHILIP RUBIN 99

14 Radiation Biocontiniuum: Follow-Up Care For Cancer Survivors:
   Needs, Issues, and Strategies
   NOREEN M. AZIZ 109

Subject Index 131

List of Contributors 127

Radiation (and Medical) Biosurveillance:

Screening Survivors for Late Effects of Therapy Using the Children's Oncology Group Long-Term Follow-Up Guidelines

Melissa M. Hudson, Wendy Landier, Smita Bhatia, Kevin C. Oeffinger, Charles Sklar, Anna Meadows, Marc Horowitz, David Poplack, Michael Fordis, and Louis S. Constine

CONTENTS

1.1 Introduction 2
1.2 Call to Action by the Institute of Medicine 2
1.3 Publication of the COG LTFU Guidelines 3
1.4 Organization of the COG LTFU Guidelines 3
1.5 Updating the COG LTFU Guidelines 4
1.6 Guideline Revisions and Enhancements 5
1.7 Passport for Care – Interactive Web-Based Version of the COG LTFU Guidelines 6
1.8 Conclusion 9
References 9

M. M. Hudson, MD
St. Jude Children's Research Hospital, Memphis, TN, USA
W. Landier, RN, MSN, CPNP, CPON
S. Bhatia, MD, MPH
City of Hope National Medical Center, Duarte, CA, USA
K. C. Oeffinger, MD
C. Sklar, MD
Memorial Sloan Kettering Cancer Center, New York, NY, USA
A. Meadows, MD
Children's Hospital of Philadelphia, Philadelphia, PA, USA
M. Horowitz, MD
D. Poplack, MD
Texas Children's Cancer Center, Houston, TX, USA
M. Fordis, MD
Baylor College of Medicine, Houston, TX, USA
L. S. Constine, MD
Department of Radiation Oncology, University of Rochester Medical Center, Rochester, NY, USA

Summary

Surveillance and management for therapy-related normal tissue damage in survivors of both childhood and adult-onset cancer is necessary to maximize health-related quality of life. Progress by the Children's Oncology Group (COG) can be modeled or adapted for adult malignancy, and is described in this report. Investigators from COG developed risk-based, exposure-related guidelines to provide recommendations for screening and management of late effects that may arise as a result of therapeutic exposures used during treatment for childhood, adolescent and young adult cancer. The guidelines are both evidence-based and grounded in the collective clinical experience of experts providing clinical care to these patient populations. A therapy-based design was chosen to permit modular formatting of the guidelines by therapeutic exposure and based on the patient's age, presenting features, and treatment era. Multidisciplinary system-based (e.g., cardiovascular, neurocognitive, reproductive, etc.) task forces organized within the COG Late Effects Committee are responsible for monitoring the literature, evaluating guideline content, and providing recommendations for guideline revision as new information becomes available. The COG Long-Term Follow-Up (LTFU) Guidelines and accompanying health education materials are available at www.survivorshipguidelines.org.

Research grant support:
This work was supported in part by the Children's Oncology Group grant U10 CA098543 from the National Cancer Institute.
Dr. Hudson is also supported by the Cancer Center Support (CORE) grant CA 21765 from the National Cancer Institute and by the American Lebanese Syrian Associated Charities (ALSAC).

1.1 Introduction

The development of curative therapy for most childhood and adolescent cancers has produced a growing population of cancer survivors who are at increased risk for a variety of late health problems resulting from their cancer or its treatment [1]. Since many treatment-related sequelae may not become clinically apparent until the survivor attains maturity or begins to age, healthcare providers need to anticipate late treatment effects in order to provide timely interventions that might prevent or correct these sequelae and their adverse effects on quality of life. Risk-based care, defined as a systematic plan for lifelong screening, surveillance, and prevention that incorporates risks based on the previous cancer, cancer therapy, genetic predispositions, lifestyle behaviors, and co-morbid health conditions, is recommended for all survivors [2, 3]. However, implementation of risk-based care for childhood cancer survivors requires a working knowledge of cancer-related health risks and appropriate screening evaluations, or access to resources containing this information. Unfortunately, most healthcare providers may be uncomfortable with managing survivors in their practice because of their lack of familiarity with the potential late effects and associated screening and counseling recommendations [4]. Motivation to gain expertise to care for this vulnerable population is hindered by the fact that the majority of providers will follow only a handful of childhood cancer survivors in their practice, all with different malignancies, treatment exposures, and healthcare risks. Addressing knowledge deficits regarding survivor care is an important public health issue; the substantial gains in years of life saved after successful therapy for a childhood or adolescent cancer will result in a significantly greater need for community-based care for adults who have survived these cancers.

In response to these concerns, investigators representing a wide range of disciplines from institutions in the Children's Oncology Group (COG) committed themselves to organizing and maintaining recommendations for screening and management of late treatment complications that could result from therapeutic exposures for childhood and adolescent cancers [5]. The resulting COG Long-Term Follow-Up Guidelines (COG LTFU Guidelines) for Survivors of Childhood, Adolescent, and Young Adult Cancers is a comprehensive educational resource available to any healthcare provider who supervises the care of a survivor of childhood cancer. The purpose of the COG LTFU Guidelines is to facilitate early identification of and intervention for treatment-related complications in order to improve quality of life for survivors with specialized healthcare needs. Herein, we briefly recount the history of the COG LTFU Guideline development previously published [5] and provide an update regarding the activities of the COG Late Effects Steering Committee and Guideline Task Forces that have contributed to assuring that the information summarized in the Guidelines meets defined criteria and is up to date.

1.2 Call to Action by the Institute of Medicine

Following the National Cancer Policy Board's meeting on childhood cancer survivorship in January 2002, the Institute of Medicine charged the COG with the development of comprehensive clinical practice guidelines for long-term follow-up care of childhood cancer survivors. The initiative began as a collaborative process between the Nursing Discipline and Late Effects Committee and subsequently expanded to involve investigators with expertise in, radiation oncology, behavioral medicine, a variety of pediatric subspecialties, and patient advocacy, in addition to nursing and pediatric oncology. Evidence collection for the guidelines involved a complete search of the medical literature for the past 20 years using MEDLINE. Keywords included "childhood cancer therapy" and "complications" combined with keywords for each therapeutic exposure. References from the bibliographies of selected articles were used to broaden the search. A multidisciplinary panel of experts in the late effects of childhood and adolescent cancer treatment reviewed and scored the guidelines using a modified version of the National Comprehensive Cancer Network "Categories of Consensus" system [6]. Each score reflects the strength of data from the literature linking a specific late effect with a therapeutic exposure, coupled with an assessment of the appropriateness of the screening recommendation based on collective clinical experience (Table 1.1). Therefore, the guidelines are both evidence-based (utilizing established associations between thera-

Table 1.1. Categories of consensus scoring for the COG LTFU guidelines

Category	Statement of consensus
1	There is uniform consensus of the panel that: (1) there is high-level evidence linking the late effect with the therapeutic exposure and (2) the screening recommendation is appropriate based on the collective clinical experience of panel members
2A	There is uniform consensus of the panel that: (1) there is lower-level evidence linking the late effect with the therapeutic exposure and (2) the screening recommendation is appropriate based on the collective clinical experience of panel members
2B	There is non-uniform consensus of the panel that: (1) there is lower-level evidence linking the late effect with the therapeutic exposure and (2) the screening recommendation is appropriate based on the collective clinical experience of panel members
3	There is major disagreement that the recommendation is appropriate

Uniform consensus, near-unanimous agreement of the panel with some possible neutral positions.
Non-uniform consensus, the majority of panel members agree with the recommendation; however, there is recognition among panel members that, given the quality of evidence, clinicians may choose to adopt different approaches.
High-level evidence, evidence derived from high quality case control or cohort studies.
Lower-level evidence, evidence derived from non-analytic studies, case reports, case series, and clinical experience.
Rather than submitting recommendations representing major disagreements, items scored as "Category 3" were either deleted or revised by the panel of experts to provide at least a "Category 2B" score for all recommendations included in the guidelines.

peutic exposures and late effects to identify high-risk categories) and grounded in the collective clinical experience of experts (matching the magnitude of the risk with the intensity of the screening recommendations).

1.3
Publication of the COG LTFU Guidelines

The Late Effects Committee released the initial version of the guidelines (Version 1.0 – Children's Oncology Group Late Effects Screening Guidelines) to the COG membership in March 2003 for a 6-month trial period to permit initial feedback in the form of targeted qualitative communications. Following additional review and revision by the Late Effects Committee, the guidelines were then released to the public (Version 1.1 – Childhood Cancer Survivor Long-Term Follow-Up Guidelines) on the COG website in September 2003. Subsequent to this release, the Late Effects Committee clarified the applicability of the guidelines to the adolescent and young adult populations of cancer survivors, which was reflected in the title change of the next guideline version (Version 1.2 – Long-Term Follow-Up Guidelines for Survivors of Childhood, Adolescent, and Young Adult Cancers) released to the public on the COG website in March 2004. Further substantial revision in both content and format of the guidelines was undertaken (Version 2.0; March 2006).

1.4
Organization of the COG LTFU Guidelines

Since therapeutic interventions for a specific childhood and adolescent cancer may vary considerably based on the patient's age, presenting features, and treatment era, a therapy-based design was chosen to permit modular formatting of the guidelines by therapeutic exposure. The screening recommendations outlined in the COG LTFU Guidelines are appropriate for asymptomatic survivors presenting for routine exposure-based medical follow-up 2 or more years after completion of therapy for a childhood, adolescent, or young adult cancer. More extensive evaluations are presumed, as clinically indicated, for survivors with signs and symptoms suggesting illness or organ dysfunction. Organization of the guidelines is summarized in Table 1.2. In addition, screening recommendations for common adult-onset secondary cancers are provided within the COG LTFU Guidelines with definitions of high-risk pop-

Table 1.2. Organization of the COG LTFU guidelines

Section number	Unique identifier for each guideline section corresponding with listing in Index
Therapeutic agent	Therapeutic intervention for malignancy, including chemotherapy, radiation, surgery, blood/serum products, hematopoietic cell transplant, and other therapeutic modalities
Potential late effects	Most common late treatment complications associated with specified therapeutic intervention
Risk factors	Host factors (e.g., age, sex, race, genetic predisposition), treatment factors (e.g., cumulative dose of therapeutic agent, mode of administration, combinations of agents), medical conditions (e.g., pre-morbid or co-morbid conditions), and health behaviors (e.g., diet, smoking, alcohol use) that may increase risk of developing the complication
Highest risk factors	Conditions (host factors, treatment factors, medical conditions, and/or health behaviors) associated with the highest risk for developing the complication
Periodic evaluations	Recommended screening evaluations, including health history, physical examination, laboratory evaluation, imaging, and psychosocial assessment. Recommendation for minimum frequency of periodic evaluations is based on risk factors and magnitude of risk, as supported by the medical literature and/or the combined clinical experience of the reviewers and panel of experts
Health counseling/ further considerations	Health Links: Health education materials developed specifically to accompany these guidelines. Title(s) of Health Link(s) relevant to each guideline section are referenced in this column. Health Link documents are included in Appendix II, and are also available on the COG website at www.survivorshipguidelines.org
	Counseling: Suggested patient counseling regarding measures to prevent/reduce risk or promote early detection of the potential treatment complication
	Resources: Books and websites that may provide the clinician with additional relevant information
	Considerations for further testing and intervention: Recommendations for further diagnostic evaluations beyond minimum screening for individuals with positive screening tests, recommendations for consultation and/or referral, and recommendations for management of exacerbating or predisposing conditions
System	Body system (e.g., auditory, musculoskeletal) most relevant to each guideline section
Score	Score assigned by expert panel representing the strength of data from the literature linking a specific late effect with a therapeutic exposure coupled with an assessment of the appropriateness of the screening recommendation based on collective clinical experience
References	References are listed immediately following each guideline section. Included are medical citations that provide evidence for the association of the therapeutic intervention with the specific treatment complication and/or evaluation of predisposing risk factors. In addition, some general review articles have been included in the Reference section for clinician convenience

ulations of childhood cancer survivors for whom heightened surveillance is recommended because of predisposing host, behavioral, or therapeutic factors (Table 1.3). Patient education materials (called "Health Links") complement a variety of survivorship topics addressed in the guidelines. The COG LTFU Guidelines and associated Health Links can be downloaded from http://www.survivorshipguidelines.org.

1.5
Updating the COG LTFU Guidelines

The COG Late Effects Committee charged 18 multidisciplinary system-based (e.g., cardiovascular, neurocognitive, fertility/reproductive, etc.) task forces with the responsibilities of monitoring the literature, evaluating guideline content, and providing recommendations for guideline revision as new informa-

Table 1.3. COG preventive screening recommendations for common adult-onset cancers

Section	Content
Organ	The organ at risk for developing malignancy
At-risk population	Populations generally considered at increased risk for the specified malignancy based on risk factors such as age, gender, genetic susceptibility, personal or family history, health-related behaviors or co-morbidities
Highest risk	Populations considered by the Panel of Experts or other evaluating bodies (such as the American Cancer Society) as being at significantly increased risk for the specified malignancy. Risk factors may include therapeutic exposures resulting from childhood cancer treatment, as well as other factors listed above (e.g., genetic susceptibility)
Periodic evaluations	Recommended screening evaluations including health history, clinical exams, laboratory evaluations, diagnostic imaging studies, psychosocial assessments, or other indicated evaluations
Standard risk	Guidelines provided under the "Standard Risk" category are per American Cancer Society recommendations for standard-risk populations and are included for clinician reference. In addition, clinicians are encouraged to consult recommendations from other organizations, such as the US Preventive Services Task Force (http://www.ahrq.gov/clinic/serfiles.htm)
Highest risk	Recommendations for high-risk populations, when applicable, are specified and may differ from recommendations for the standard-risk groups due to the significantly increased risk of the specified malignancy within the high-risk group

tion becomes available. Each guideline task force recruited representatives from nursing, pediatric oncology, radiation oncology, primary care, patient advocacy and pediatric/medical subspecialty care, as appropriate. Specific task force responsibilities include preparation and presentation of a bi-annual report to the Late Effects Committee that: (1) summarizes new literature related to the task force topic; (2) clarifies unfamiliar terms in the guideline content that could be misinterpreted; and (3) provides recommendations with rationale for guideline revisions. The task forces have already contributed innumerable hours of time and effort that are reflected in the revisions and refinements of each version of the guidelines. Many task force members are also pursuing other scholarly activities in order to disseminate information about risk-based childhood cancer survivor care or address knowledge deficits identified in the organization of the COG LTFU Guidelines. These include the development of manuscripts targeting primary and subspecialty care providers, organization of research initiatives, and educational presentations in various community and academic forums. These efforts are anticipated to facilitate the goals of the COG LTFU Guidelines to educate healthcare providers and patients about late effects and standardize and enhance follow-up care of childhood and adolescent cancer survivors.

1.6
Guideline Revisions and Enhancements

Following their organization, the guideline task forces undertook a thorough review of the literature used to derive the original guideline recommendations, as well as new publications relevant to the task force topic. The Late Effects Steering Committee assigned guideline sections to task forces based on established associations with specific treatment exposures and potential late effects (e.g., the Fertility/Reproductive Task Force was assigned to review literature relevant to alkylating agent chemotherapy and gonadal dysfunction). Each task force organized the results of its review in a summary report accompanied by a comprehensive Late Effects Evidence Table outlining the Medline citation, type of study (systematic review, meta analysis, randomized control trial, nonrandomized control trial, observational study, non-experimental studies, expert opinion, general review), number of patients participating in study/cohort, study objective(s), and brief summary of study findings. In the summary report, findings of the literature review were categorized as "confirmatory" if supportive of findings of previous publications; "disputable" if contrary to findings of previous publications; or "novel" if not previously reported. The reports emphasized association(s) of therapeutic exposure(s) and late effect(s), defined risk factors for late effects, and detailed recommendations for specific screening test(s) for a given late effect. Task force recommendations for guideline revisions were then presented to the Late Effects Steering Committee for approval and scoring before incorporation into the COG LTFU Guidelines.

The recently published Version 2.0 features extensive revisions in content that reflect enhanced clinical (particularly subspecialty) expertise in guideline task force membership that facilitated more prudent interpretation of findings from the medical literature, definition of risk groups, and assignment of screening recommendations. A total of 34 new therapeutic exposures were added, including specific sections for complications associated with total body irradiation and hematopoietic cell transplant, as well as hematopoietic cell transplant with chronic graft-versus-host-disease. Sections related to systemic radiation (e.g., MIBG) and bioimmunotherapy (e.g., granulocyte-colony stimulating factor) treatments were also added as the populations of childhood cancer survivors treated with these relatively novel approaches are now increasing in numbers. The radiation treatment sections in Version 2.0, one of the most substantially revised topic areas, now include sections delineated by both dose and volume with impact to specific target organs, e.g., brain/cranium, neuroendocrine axis, thyroid, heart, lungs, and other organs. In addition, many of the representative citations have been revised to provide clinicians with references that reflect the depth and/or breadth of evidence in the literature that support specific guideline recommendations. Finally, nine new Health Links have been developed to address topics meriting patient education materials and all of the Health Links have been updated to reflect new guideline recommendations and to improve readability.

Version 2.0 also features a variety of new resources to assist clinicians who may be unfamiliar with some of the technical terms related to childhood cancer survivor care. These include appendices with summary tables outlining abbreviations appearing in the guidelines, generic and brand names of chemotherapeutic agents, and definitions of standardly used radiation treatment fields. A cancer treatment summary is required in order to interface with the COG LTFU Guidelines and determine the recommended follow-up care for individual survivors. To facilitate implementation of the COG LTFU Guidelines, Version 2.0 provides appendices outlining the essential elements of a Cancer Treatment Summary, as well as a Guideline Identification Tool that links specific treatment exposures with corresponding guideline sections (Fig. 1.1). Language and abbreviations throughout the Guidelines have also been standardized in preparation for a computerized, web-based guideline generator (see Sect. 1.7). To enhance readability for the numerous clinicians and survivors accessing the guidelines through http://www.survivorshipguidelines.org, substantial changes have also been undertaken in the layout, format, and font of the document. Figure 1.2 provides a sample illustration of the new content and format in Version 2.0 of the guidelines.

1.7
Passport for Care – Interactive Web-Based Version of the COG LTFU Guidelines

The current format of the COG LTFU Guidelines poses significant barriers to routine use by busy clinicians due to their volume and density. Presently, the COG LTFU Guidelines are comprised of 145 sections of detailed evidence-based recommendations encompassing 175 pages, not including the introductory materials, appendices, and index. While specific supporting health education materials that are pertinent to therapeutic exposures and provide recommendations for a given patient are available as separate documents with easy downloading and printing, the provider must currently locate all guideline sections applicable to each survivor within the lengthy document. A computerized, interactive version of the guidelines will facilitate rapid identification of specific recommendations pertinent to the care of an individual patient, substantially expediting implementation of risk-based childhood cancer survivor care as outlined by the COG LTFU Guidelines.

Through collaboration of investigators from COG Late Effects Committee, Texas Children's Cancer

Fig. 1.1. Page 1 of *Patient-Specific Guideline Identification Tool*, which outlines the essential elements of a cancer treatment summary and links specific treatment exposures with corresponding guideline sections

CureSearch
Children's Oncology Group

Patient-Specific Guideline Identification Tool
(Applicable Guideline Sections indicated in Bold/Red; M = Male; F = Female)

Name:	Sex: M/F	Date of Birth:

Cancer Diagnosis: _____	Date of Diagnosis: _____	End Therapy Date: _____
☑ Sections 1 & 2 applicable to all patients	Prior to 1972: ☐ Section 3 Prior to 1993: ☐ Section 4 1977 - 1985: ☐ Section 5	LTFU guidelines are applicable to patients who are ≥2 years following completion of cancer therapy

CHEMOTHERAPY: ☐ Yes ☐ No If yes: ☑ Section 6 and applicable guidelines for specific chemotherapy agents below

Chemotherapy Agent (✓ if patient received)	Applicable guideline sections	
Asparaginase	Section 34	
Bleomycin	Section 29	
Busulfan	Sections 7M/F, 8, 9, 10	
Carboplatin – all doses	Sections 7M/F, 8, 15, 16, 17	
– myeloablative dose	See also: Section 14	Note: Myeloablative dose = conditioning for HCT
Carmustine	Sections 7M/F, 8, 9	
Chlorambucil	Sections 7M/F, 8	
Cisplatin	Sections 7M/F, 8, 14, 15, 16, 17	
Cyclophosphamide	Sections 7M/F, 8, 11, 12	
Cytarabine: SQ, IT, IO, low-dose IV	Section 20	Note: Low-dose IV = all single doses < 1000 mg/m^2
Cytarabine: High-dose IV	Sections 18, 19	Note: High-dose IV = any single dose ≥1000 mg/m^2
Dacarbazine	Sections 7M/F, 8	
Dactinomycin	Section 30	
Daunorubicin Cumulative dose: _____ mg/m^2 Age at first dose: _____	Sections 27, 28	
Dexamethasone	Sections 31, 32, 33	
Doxorubicin Cumulative dose: _____ mg/m^2 Age at first dose: _____	Sections 27, 28	
Epirubicin* Cumulative dose: _____ mg/m^2 Age at first dose: _____	Sections 27, 28 Cumulative dose x 0.67 = _____ mg/m^2 = doxorubicin/daunorubicin isotoxic dose	
Etoposide (VP-16)	Section 37	
Idarubicin* Cumulative dose: _____ mg/m^2 Age at first dose: _____	Sections 27, 28 Cumulative dose x 5 = _____ mg/m^2 = doxorubicin/daunorubicin isotoxic dose	
Ifosfamide	Sections 7M/F, 8, 11, 13	
Lomustine	Sections 7M/F, 8, 9	
Mechlorethamine	Sections 7M/F, 8	
Melphalan	Sections 7M/F, 8	
Mercaptopurine (6-MP)	Section 21	

*Use formulas below to convert to doxorubicin/daunorubicin isotoxic equivalents prior to calculating total cumulative anthracycline dose:
Epirubicin - multiply total dose x 0.67   **Idarubicin** - multiply total dose x 5   **Mitoxantrone** - multiply total dose x 3.5
Note: There is a paucity of literature to support isotoxic dose conversion; however, the above conversion factors may be used for convenience in order to gauge screening frequency. Clinical judgment should ultimately be used to determine indicated screening for individual patients.

RADIATION

Sec #	Therapeutic Agent(s)	Potential Late Effects	Risk Factors	Highest Risk Factors	Periodic Evaluation	Health Counseling Further Considerations
68 (Female)	≥ 20 Gy to: Mantle Mini-Mantle Mediastinal Chest (thorax) Axilla	Breast cancer	**Host Factors** Family history of breast cancer **Treatment Factors** Higher radiation dose Longer time since radiation (≥ 5 years) **Info Link** There is currently a deficiency in the literature regarding whether or not TBI is a risk factor for the development of breast cancer. Monitoring of patients who received TBI should be determined on an individual basis.	**Host Factors** Female gender	**PHYSICAL** Breast exam (Yearly beginning at puberty until age 25, then every six months) **SCREENING** Mammogram (Beginning 8 years after radiation or at age 25, whichever occurs last) **Info Link**: Mammography is currently limited in its ability to evaluate the premenopausal breast. The role of MRI is evolving for screening of other populations at high risk for breast cancer (e.g., premenopausal known or likely carriers of gene mutation of known penetrance).	**Health Links** Breast Cancer **Counseling** Teach breast self-exam and counsel to perform monthly beginning at puberty. **Considerations for Further Testing and Intervention** Surgical consultation for diagnostic procedure in patients with breast mass or suspicious radiographic finding. Decisions regarding the use of HRT should be based on current literature and should take into consideration the risk/benefit ratio for individual patients. SYSTEM = SMN SCORE = 1

POTENTIAL IMPACT TO BREAST

SECTION 68 REFERENCES

Bhatia S, Robison LL, Oberlin O, et al. Breast cancer and other second neoplasms after childhood Hodgkin's disease. *N Engl J Med.* Mar 21 1996;334(12):745-751.
Bhatia S, Yasui Y, Robison LL, et al. High risk of subsequent neoplasms continues with extended follow-up of childhood Hodgkin's disease: report from the Late Effects Study Group. *J Clin Oncol.* Dec 1 2003;21(23):4386-4394.
Goss PE, Sierra S. Current perspectives on radiation-induced breast cancer. *J Clin Oncol.* Jan 1998;16(1):338-347.
Guibout C, Adjadj E, Rubino C, et al. Malignant breast tumors after radiotherapy for a first cancer during childhood. *J Clin Oncol.* Jan 1 2005;23(1):197-204.
Kaste SC, Hudson MM, Jones DJ, et al. Breast masses in women treated for childhood cancer: incidence and screening guidelines. *Cancer.* Feb 15 1998;82(4):784-792.
Kenney LB, Yasui Y, Inskip PD, et al. Breast cancer after childhood cancer: a report from the Childhood Cancer Survivor Study. *Ann Intern Med.* Oct 19 2004;141(8):590-597.
Metayer C, Lynch CF, Clarke EA, et al. Second cancers among long-term survivors of Hodgkin's disease diagnosed in childhood and adolescence. *J Clin Oncol.* Jun 2000;18(12):2435-2443.
Travis LB, Hill DA, Dores GM, et al. Breast cancer following radiotherapy and chemotherapy among young women with Hodgkin disease. *JAMA.* Jul 23 2003;290(4):465-475.
van Leeuwen FE, Klokman WJ, Stovall M, et al. Roles of radiation dose, chemotherapy, and hormonal factors in breast cancer following Hodgkin's disease. *J Natl Cancer Inst.* Jul 2 2003;95(13):971-980.
Wolden SL, Hancock SL, Carlson RW, Goffinet DR, Jeffrey SS, Hoppe RT. Management of breast cancer after Hodgkin's disease. *J Clin Oncol.* Feb 2000;18(4):765-772.

Version 2.0 – March 2006

Fig. 1.2. Sample illustration of the new content and format in Version 2.0 of the COG Long-Term Follow-Up Guidelines (COG LTFU Guidelines) for Survivors of Childhood, Adolescent, and Young Adult Cancers featuring the potential late effect of breast cancer after radiation and the recommended surveillance

Center, and Baylor College of Medicine, significant progress has been made in developing an interactive web-based version of the COG LTFU Guidelines. This online decision support tool, known as Passport for Care, will permit healthcare providers and childhood cancer survivors to quickly and accurately generate individualized exposure-based screening recommendations and patient educational materials according to the COG LTFU- Guidelines. The web-based, user-friendly interface includes a cancer treatment summary form that allows streamlined entry of key patient data (e.g., therapeutic exposures, cumulative doses for selected agents) in order to generate individualized follow-up recommendations. The Passport for Care also provides the COG Late Effects Committee with a set of online tools and reports to facilitate guideline development, review, editing, and updating for purposes of maintaining guideline standardization and consistency. Standardization of the content and format undertaken in COG LTFU Guidelines Version 2.0 represents a critical step before implementation of the planned testing of the Passport for Care Guideline Generator in pilot institutions in the near future.

1.8 Conclusion

Investigators with expertise in many areas participating in the COG LTFU Guideline Task Forces have produced a comprehensive and dynamic resource that provides practical recommendations for evaluation and management of late effects in childhood cancer survivors. The COG LTFU Guidelines aim to enhance providers' familiarity regarding the special healthcare needs of this vulnerable and growing population, and facilitate risk-based screening for cancer-related late treatment complications. The Late Effects Committee and LTFU Guideline Task Forces' ongoing maintenance and dissemination efforts in information relevant to survivor health and research initiatives addressing knowledge deficits about cancer treatment effects provides strong support of the COG's commitment to long-term survivor health. Strategies such as Passport for Care, that can efficiently disseminate targeted information, will be critical to the integration of the guideline recommendations in routine survivor care in a primary care setting. The strategy of guideline development and refinement used by the COG may be adapted by clinicians supervising the care of survivors of adult malignancies who encounter health risks after cancer treatment.

Acknowledgements

The authors would like to thank the many individuals participating in the COG Guideline Task Forces who have dedicated their time and expertise to the COG LTFU Guideline development and maintenance.

References

1. Hewitt M, Weiner SL, Simone JV (eds) (2003) Childhood cancer survivorship: improving care and quality of life. National Cancer Policy Board, Washington, D.C
2. Oeffinger KC (2003) Longitudinal risk-based health care for adult survivors of childhood cancer. Curr Probl Cancer 27:143–167
3. Oeffinger KC, Hudson MM (2004) Long-term complications following childhood and adolescent cancer: foundations for providing risk-based health care for survivors. CA Cancer J Clin 54:208–236
4. Landier W, Wallace WH, Hudson MM (2006) Long-term follow-up of pediatric cancer survivors: education, surveillance, and screening. Pediatr Blood Cancer 46:149–158
5. Landier W, Bhatia S, Eshelman DA et al (2004) Development of risk-based guidelines for pediatric cancer survivors: the Children's Oncology Group Long-Term Follow-Up Guidelines from the Children's Oncology Group Late Effects Committee and Nursing Discipline. J Clin Oncol 22:4979–4990
6. Winn RJ, Botnick WZ (1997) The NCCN Guideline Program: a conceptual framework. Oncology (Williston Park) 11:25–32

Medical Countermeasures to Radiation Injury: Science and Service in the Public Interest

Tribute to Robert Kallman, LENT V meeting 2004

C. NORMAN COLEMAN

CONTENTS

2.1 Introduction 11
2.1.1 Contributions of Dr. Kallman and Colleagues: Science and Service 12

2.2 Radiation Biology and Medical Countermeasures to Radiation 13

2.3 Mechanisms and Models 15

2.4 Conclusions and Future Directions 15

References 16

Presented in part at the Late Effects Normal Tissues (LENT V) meeting, Rochester, NY, May 23–25, 2004.
The content and opinions within this manuscript are from the author and not the US Government.

C. N. COLEMAN, MD
Associate Director, Radiation Research Program, EPN/Room 6014, 6130 Executive Boulevard, Bethesda, MD 20892, USA

Summary

Radiation oncologists, biologists, epidemiologists, and health physicists have a long-standing interest in understanding the risk, etiology, prevention, and treatment of radiation damage to normal tissue as a consequence of exposure of healthy populations, as well as from cancer treatment. The recent threat of radiological and nuclear terrorism as a consequence of a radiological dispersion device (RDD) or improvised nuclear device (IND) has raised public awareness of the consequences of radiation exposure. Normal tissue injury results from local cellular and tissue processes directly damaged by the radiation, as well as from the response of the entire organism. The development of effective medical countermeasures to protect, mitigate, and/or treat normal tissue injury requires investigation from basic molecular mechanisms to multicellular systems to relevant animal models to clinical trials. With renewed interest and support, the radiation biology/oncology research community has a critical opportunity for scientific investigation and service to society by advancing knowledge, helping oncology patients, and enhancing the well-being of entire populations living under the threat of accidental or intentional radiation exposure.

2.1 Introduction

The Late Effects Normal Tissues (LENT) V meeting honored the contributions of the late Dr. Robert Kallman of the Stanford Department of Radiation Oncology. In that I had the opportunity to be a student and colleague of his and a friend to him and his wife, Ingrid, who graciously attended the meeting, this paper is a tribute to his contributions and a personal perspective of their direct relevance to the field of normal tissue biology addressed at this meeting. The theme of this paper, and indeed a sub-theme of the LENT V meeting, is the importance of planning and conducting scientific experimentation with an eye to both new knowledge and public service. Science contributes a great deal to society in the US and society contributes a great deal to the support of science through financial investment, prestige afforded scientists and physicians, and advocacy for the free and open pursuit of knowledge. Knowledge for its own sake is an extraordinarily valuable contribution, yet there are times when the need for new knowledge and public service in a field coincide.

2.1.1
Contributions of Dr. Kallman and Colleagues: Science and Service

Borne from technology and nuclear physics of World War II, the 1950–60s was an era of great advances for radiation biology and oncology resulting from technological advances in radar (klystrons) and electronics, leading to the development of the clinical linear accelerator, and to the advent of cell culture techniques by which to study cell survival curves following radiation and/or drug treatment. Of paramount importance was the public health necessity to learn about the effects of nuclear exposure to people as the world entered the atomic era and the threat of further nuclear warfare.

Starting in the 1950s, the Stanford University Department of Radiology became a world leader in radiation oncology and biology research. Dr. Henry S. Kaplan was a true giant in making radiation oncology into a science-based discipline and distinguishing its clinical application from that of diagnostic radiology in which it was embedded [1]. Dr. Kaplan's substantial laboratory discoveries, including the viral etiology of mouse leukemia and the laboratory and clinical investigation of the human lymphomas, accompanied his efforts toward the development of the first clinical linear accelerator in the US [2, 3] and the curative treatment of Hodgkin's disease [4]. Drs. Kaplan and Saul Rosenberg recognized the critical importance of science-based and, indeed, evidence-based clinical medicine. Under Dr. Kaplan's overall departmental leadership, Dr. Kallman was instrumental in building and leading a world renowned radiation and cancer biology program.

During my decade at Stanford (1975–1985), the Division of Radiation Biology included Drs. Bob Kallman, Kendric Smith, George Hahn, and Martin Brown, representing a spectrum of expertise from DNA repair to cellular and tissue radiation biology, to radiation–drug interactions, to hyperthermia biology and treatment, to hypoxia, and to radiation sensitizers and protectors. Dr. Luis Fajardo's expertise in radiation pathology [5, 6] brought further mechanistic information to pioneering work by Dr. Philip Rubin [7], one of the leaders of this LENT V conference and a long-standing force behind the field of radiation toxicity. For those fortunate to be at Stanford during these years, a critical theme of the leadership of Drs. Kaplan, Rosenberg, and Bagshaw was the linkage between laboratory investigation and human application.

Dr. Kallman's research in radiation biology and in radiation–drug interaction [8–11] are relevant to today's research in combined modality therapy, normal tissue injury, and lethality following whole body radiation exposure [12, 13]. The period of rapid growth of radiation biology was followed by a period of stability and then decline in investment in this field. The establishment of the specialty of medical oncology led to a focus in cancer research on drug development and the growth in complexity of radiation technology and instrumentation diverted attention and resources of the clinical departments from radiation biology to medical physics. While such investment in radiation technology was logical and important, there was a perception among laboratory-based radiation oncology physician-scientists of a decreased investment in faculty who conducted basic and translational radiobiology research. The end of the cold war lessened the perception of a threat from nuclear energy, although the occasional nuclear accident reminded the world of the need to understand radiation injury and carcinogenesis and to prevent or treat them.

Following September 11, 2001, the world has awoken to the constant anxiety of exposure to radiation from a radiological dispersion device (RDD), including a "dirty bomb" or other environmental contamination, and from an improvised nuclear device (IND) which involves a nuclear detonation. The need for information, knowledge, and research from the radiation biology and oncology communities was immediately apparent.

2.2 Radiation Biology and Medical Countermeasures to Radiation

Normal tissue injury is an essential component of the practice of clinical radiation oncology. Radiation protectors have been an interest for many years with amifostine currently in clinical use [14] for salivary gland protection. Other indications such as mucosal protection are being further investigated, as is the subcutaneous route of administration which appears to be better tolerated than the intravenous route [15, 16] yet equally effective in the laboratory [17].

Improved technology for radiation therapy allows for the delivery of a higher tumor dose. Nonetheless, normal tissue toxicity will still limit the delivery of a tumoricidal dose as recent studies of late effects indicate [18, 19]. Furthermore, combined modality therapy may produce an enhanced injury profile as seen with newly described consequential late effects [20]. While allowing dose escalation to and within a tumor, intensity modulated radiation therapy (IMRT) has a potential drawback of exposing more normal tissue to some dose compared to 3D-conformal treatments, potentially increasing the carcinogenicity of treatment [21, 22]. The low dose but relatively high volume exposure of normal tissue may have relevance to non-oncology populations subject to accidental or intentional radiation exposure. Thus, there is much that can be learned from clinical radiation therapy applicable to population exposure to ionizing radiation.

The NCI Radiation Research Program (RRP) has conducted a number of workshops related to normal tissue injury (Table 2.1).

Table 2.1. Radiation Research Program workshops

Normal tissue injury, 2000 [23]
Moderate dose radiation, 2001 [30]
Clinical Common Toxicity Criteria (CTCAE3.0), 2002 [32]
Radiation Biology Education and Training, 2003 [33]
Normal tissue, animal models, 2003 [53]
Normal tissue, animal models, preclinical emphasis, 2004 (NIAID/NCI)
Workshops under discussion by NIAID/NCI include, among others: partial body exposure, carcinogenesis, biodosimetry

The Normal Tissue Injury workshop in 2000 [23] brought together experts from radiation biology, imaging, and wound healing, recognizing the similarities between general tissue injury and that related to radiation. Clinical reports demonstrating that the manifestations of late normal tissue injury may be reversible [24–26] support the model that radiation damage is a dynamic process involving ongoing tissue injury. Consequently, while pre-exposure treatment remains critical to avoiding and preventing injury, post-exposure intervention is a strategy to pursue for clinical and population exposure [27, 28].

Shortly after September 11th, the specter of an RDD or IND led the RRP and colleagues from the radiation research community to conduct a workshop on what we defined as moderate dose radiation, that is, 1–10 Gy in either a single or fractionated dose. This dose was chosen for the following reasons: (a) very low dose exposure (< 0.1 Gy) is actively being investigated by the Department of Energy (DOE); (b) gene induction following radiation occurs at 1 Gy and even at lower doses making it likely that there will be measurable effects for which modulating agents can be tested [29]; (c) in whole body exposure, this dose range will produce the hematopoietic and gastrointestinal syndromes, both of which require clinical intervention [30]; (d) IMRT will produce doses in this range to a wide array of normal tissues [21] so that clinical investigation could be accomplished in radiation oncology that would pertain to people subject to accidental or intentional exposure; (e) such doses are carcinogenic [22, 31]; and (f) there was limited clinical and preclinical investigation ongoing in this moderate dose range. This meeting helped define the current state of the science and opportunities in: basic research, technology development, particularly for biodosimetry; treatment strategies; and ensuring sufficient expertise in radiation biology and related sciences [30].

The Cancer Treatment Evaluation Program (CTEP) continually refines and updates standards and methodology for clinical trials including the development of toxicity criteria. As part of an ongoing effort to further define late effects, an updated system, Common Toxicity Criteria for Adverse Events (CTCAEv3.0) [32] has been established that brings together a number of systems into one common system. In that the spectrum of tissue injury may reflect both the high and lower dose exposures, having a clinical scoring system by which radiation modifiers can be judged will allow the study of such protectors, mitigators, and treatments to be used in oncology trials. Of course, the issue of tumor protection must be considered for oncology. For practice and research in oncology and for addressing radiation exposure in the general population, a clinically validated scoring system is of great value. Further work is ongoing to develop a hand-held device for clinical use that makes this complex system more user-friendly and available for use in the clinic and field (Trotti, personal communication).

Essential to the research and development effort is the need for trained scientists and other personnel, an issue addressed by the The Education and Training Workshop [33]. The immediate focus is on developing doctoral training programs in radiation biology. Postdoctoral training and collaboration among radiation biologists and between radiation biologists and other scientists will help stimulate research and also help recruit new people to the field. A Council for Radiation Research Societies was suggested to enhance coordination among nongovernmental agencies (Radiation Research Society, American Society of Therapeutic Radiology and Oncology, American Association of Physicists in Medicine, American College or Radiology, and others). This complements an informal interagency collaborative group Radiation Bioterrorism Research and Training (RABRAT) that is ongoing among Federal agencies [33].

Developing effective clinical interventions requires appropriate model systems addressed in an Animal Models workshop in 2004 [34]. Figure 2.1 illustrates the range of systems needed, the goal of which is to bring scientific discovery to people. Normal tissue injury involves damage and response from the molecular, cellular, tissue, and organism level so that a full range of models is needed. Novel model systems include multicellular systems, yeast, *C. elegans* and Zebrafish. Preclinical testing requires larger species. Although it may not be possible to validate the effectiveness of a radiation countermeasure in a clinical trial, phase I trials are necessary for FDA approval (under the "animal rule" – see FDA website). In this regard, radiation countermeasures may not only help oncology patients but the ability to assess the efficacy in addition to the safety of new agents in the clinic provides a unique and essential role for radiation oncology translational research in the development of medical countermeasures for radiation.

A new program for Federal support for research related to radiological/nuclear terrorism is channeled through Health and Human Services (HHS) via the National Institute for Allergy and Infectious Diseases (NIAID), in collaboration with NCI. A second normal tissue workshop was held addressing animal models with an emphasis on preclinical development (May, 2004). As noted in Table 2.1, additional workshops are under consideration for addressing effects of partial body exposure as the result of shielding, carcinogenesis, and biodosimetry (February, 2005).

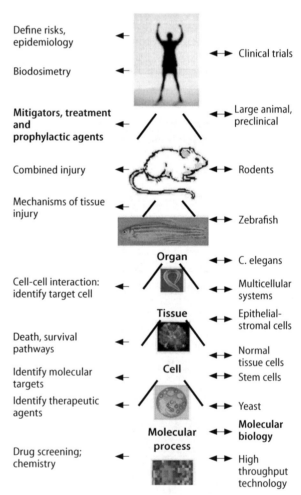

Fig. 2.1. Animal models for radiation countermeasures research. The overall goal of research is to go from underlying molecular mechanism to human application. This requires many model systems. (Adapted and reprinted with permission from [34])

2.3 Mechanisms and Models

The LENT V meeting and previous workshops noted above have described a range of potential targets and mechanisms for radiation countermeasures. A number of approaches that are in clinical use address free radical mechanisms, including amifostine [35, 36] and tempol [37, 38], which are examples of prophylactic or preventive agents given before radiation. Angiotensin converting enzyme (ACE) and Angiotensin II (AII) receptor antagonists, which have been shown to reduce radiation injury to the kidney following whole body radiation for bone marrow transplantation, are examples of radiation mitigators [39, 40]. Pentoxyfylline has been shown to be effective in the treatment of existing radiation injury [25, 26, 41]. Thus, there are model systems addressing the concepts of prevention/prophylaxis (pre-exposure), mitigation (post-exposure to reduce effect) and treatment (post-exposure to treat functional abnormality), terms that have historically been lumped under radiation protectors [34].

Three new molecular targets are described below as examples of new discoveries and also to emphasize the need for relevant model systems for the moderate dose range.

p53 can lead to apoptosis or cell cycle arrest. Komarov demonstrated that a small molecule inhibitor of p53 could protect mice against death following irradiation [42]. Further work demonstrated that protection occurs at doses that produce bone marrow death by preventing apoptosis; however, at higher radiation doses where gastrointestinal death occurs, the p53 inhibitors actually enhanced toxicity by preventing cell cycle arrest and subsequent repair [43, 44]. Of interest, when the higher dose was given as fractionated radiation rather than a single dose, protection was again seen [44]. Thus, the efficacy of this approach depends on target organ, radiation dose, and fractionation.

Ceramide-induced apoptosis has been modified using mice with a knock out of acid sphingomyelinase, such that apoptosis is reduced. At a single large radiation dose that causes gastrointestinal damage, the critical target cell for intestinal injury was the endothelial cell and not the epithelial cell [45]. What happens at fractionated doses remains to be determined.

TGFβ and SMAD signaling are involved in tissue fibrosis. Their complex mechanisms of activation and action [28, 46] provide a range of potential targets. For example, inhibiting activation with Type II receptor antagonists reduces the extent of radiation fibrosis in mice [47, 48] as does inhibition with the small molecule halofuginone [49].

The above examples, as well as other approaches under investigation [30, 50] demonstrate that there are both existing countermeasures available and novel ideas being developed. The hematopoietic cytokines and epithelial growth factors are also potential post-exposure treatments for the acute radiation syndromes [51, 52].

2.4 Conclusions and Future Directions

As a consequence of circumstances unthinkable just a few years ago, the fields of radiation biology, oncology, epidemiology, health physics, and related sciences have an opportunity and obligation to bring our expertise to bear on the needs of the society from which we derive our support. There is expertise needed from the basic mechanisms of cellular injury and that of short- and long-term tissue injury, to translational laboratory models, to clinical development, to epidemiology, to education and training and to being a part of a community medical response team. The knowledge that arises and the interventions that emerge will bring first-rate scientific discovery to the prevention, mitigation, and treatment of radiation injury to healthy populations with the potential for use in cancer treatment.

Fortunately, as illustrated in the LENT V conference, there is a cadre of scientists pursuing this area of investigation so that the understanding of radiation injury at the molecular, cellular, tissue, and organism level has increased substantially in recent years. The Federal Government is implementing a program through Health and Human Services, NIAID (http://www2.niaid.nih.gov/biodefense/) and NCI to support the development of medical interventions. This program will support Centers for Medical Countermeasures against Radiation (CMCR), special projects and product development. It will support education and training to replenish the field of radiation biology and it will be built on a strongly collaborative model to speed the development of effective countermeasures for radiation injury to clinical application.

Returning to the legacy of Dr. Robert Kallman, Dr. Henry Kaplan and their colleagues, the field of radiation biology has its underpinnings in addressing human health issues and has a long-standing tradition of conducting high quality science in the public interest. The circumstances we now face and the challenges thrust upon us require teamwork, collaboration, innovation, focus, and critical assessment of products to help populations worldwide deal with medical consequences of exposure to ionizing radiation. The common goals are through new and existing knowledge to develop methods of prevention, mitigation, treatment, and, equally important, to provide guidance and assurance to the public based on well-founded knowledge.

Note Added in Proof

The CMCR program is now in its first year under the leadership of NIAID with input from NCI. The awardees (and PI) are (alphabetically): Columbia University (David Brenner), Dana Farber Cancer Center (Alan D'Andrea), Duke University (Nelson Chao), Fred Hutchinson Cancer Center (George Georges), Medical College of Wisconsin (John Moulder), University of California, Los Angeles (William McBride), University of Pittsburgh (Joel Greenberger), and University of Rochester (Paul Okunieff). Additional workshops and meetings have been held or are in progress involving multiple federal agencies and scientists from the public and private sectors on topics including biodosimetry, medical countermeasure development and education/training. Expert system-based medical guidelines for managing a radiological/nuclear event are in preparation in the Radiological Events Medical Management (REMM) program developed by the Office of Public Health Emergency Preparedness and National Library of Medicine.

References

1. Bagshaw MA, Kallman RF, Rubin P (1985) In memoriam. Henry Seymour Kaplan. Int J Radiat Oncol Biol Phys 11:1–3
2. Kaplan HS, Bagshaw MA (1957) The Stanford medical linear accelerator. III. Application to clinical problems of radiation therapy. Stanford Med Bull 15:141–151
3. Ginzton EL, Nunan CS (1985) History of microwave electron linear accelerators for radiotherapy. Int J Radiat Oncol Biol Phys 11:205–216
4. Rosenberg SA, Kaplan HS (1985) The evolution and summary results of the Stanford randomized clinical trials of the management of Hodgkin's disease: 1962–1984. Int J Radiat Oncol Biol Phys 11:5–22
5. Fajardo LF, Stewart JR, Cohn KE (1968) Morphology of radiation-induced heart disease. Arch Pathol 86:512–519
6. Fajardo LF, Brown JM, Glatstein E (1976) Glomerular and juxta-glomerular lesions in radiation nephropathy. Radiat Res 68:177–183
7. Rubin P, Casarett GW (1968) Clinical radiation pathology as applied to curative radiotherapy. Cancer 22:767–778
8. Kallman RF, Silini G, Van Putten LM (1967) Factors influencing the quantitative estimation of the in vivo survival of cells from solid tumors. J Natl Cancer Inst 39:539–549
9. Kallman RF, Rapacchietta D, Zaghloul MS (1991) Schedule-dependent therapeutic gain from the combination of fractionated irradiation plus c-DDP and 5-FU or plus c-DDP and cyclophosphamide in C3H/Km mouse model systems. Int J Radiat Oncol Biol Phys 20:227–232
10. Kallman RF (1975) Animal experiments in radiotherapy I - small animals. J Can Assoc Radiol 26:15–24
11. Kallman RF (1963) Recovery from radiation injury: a proposed mechanism. Nature 197:557–560
12. Kallman RF, Silini G, Taylor HM 3rd (1966) Recuperation from lethal injury by whole-body irradiation. II. Kinetic aspects in radiosensitive BALB-c mice, and cyclic fine structure during the four days after conditioning irradiation. Radiat Res 29:362–394
13. Kallman RF, Silini G (1964) Recuperation from lethal injury by whole-body irradiation. I. Kinetic aspects and the relationship with conditioning dose in C57bl mice. Radiat Res 22:622–642
14. Curran W (2002) The first investigators' congress on radioprotection. Semin Radiat Oncol 12:1–111
15. Penz M, Kornek GV, Raderer M et al (2001) Subcutaneous administration of amifostine: a promising therapeutic option in patients with oxaliplatin-related peripheral sensitive neuropathy. Ann Oncol 12:421–422
16. Koukourakis MI, Simopoulos C, Minopoulos G et al (2003) Amifostine before chemotherapy: improved tolerance profile of the subcutaneous over the intravenous route. Clin Cancer Res 9:3288–3293
17. Cassatt DR, Fazenbaker CA, Kifle G et al (2003) Subcutaneous administration of amifostine (ethyol) is equivalent to intravenous administration in a rat mucositis model. Int J Radiat Oncol Biol Phys 57:794–802
18. Miller KL, Shafman TD, Anscher MS et al (2005) Bronchial stenosis: an underreported complication of high-dose external beam radiotherapy for lung cancer? Int J Radiat Oncol Biol Phys 61:64–69
19. Stripp D, Glatstein E (2005) The good, the bad, and the ugly. Int J Radiat Oncol Biol Phys 61:3–4
20. Dorr W, Hendry JH (2001) Consequential late effects in normal tissues. Radiother Oncol 61:223–231
21. Followill D, Geis P, Boyer A (1997) Estimates of whole-body dose equivalent produced by beam intensity modulated conformal therapy. Int J Radiat Oncol Biol Phys 38:667–672
22. Hall EJ, Wuu CS (2003) Radiation-induced second cancers: the impact of 3D-CRT and IMRT. Int J Radiat Oncol Biol Phys 56:83–88
23. Stone HB, McBride WH, Coleman CN (2002) Modifying normal tissue damage postirradiation. Report of a work-

shop sponsored by the Radiation Research Program, National Cancer Institute, Bethesda, Maryland, September 6–8, 2000. Radiat Res 157:204–223
24. Delanian S, Balla-Mekias S, Lefaix JL (1999) Striking regression of chronic radiotherapy damage in a clinical trial of combined pentoxifylline and tocopherol. J Clin Oncol 17:3283–3290
25. Okunieff P, Augustine E, Hicks JE et al (2004) Pentoxifylline in the treatment of radiation-induced fibrosis. J Clin Oncol 22:2207–2213
26. Delanian S, Porcher R, Balla-Mekias S, et al (2003) Randomized, placebo-controlled trial of combined pentoxifylline and tocopherol for regression of superficial radiation-induced fibrosis. J Clin Oncol 21:2545–2550
27. Rubin P, Johnston CJ, Williams JP et al (1995) A perpetual cascade of cytokines postirradiation leads to pulmonary fibrosis. Int J Radiat Oncol Biol Phys 33:99–109
28. Martin M, Lefaix J, Delanian S (2000) TGF-beta 1 and radiation fibrosis: a master switch and a specific therapeutic target? Int J Radiat Oncol Biol Phys 47:277–290
29. Amundson SA, Bittner M, Meltzer P et al (2001) Induction of gene expression as a monitor of exposure to ionizing radiation. Radiat Res 156:657–661
30. Coleman CN, Blakely WF, Fike JR et al (2003) Molecular and cellular biology of moderate-dose (1–10 Gy) radiation and potential mechanisms of radiation protection: report of a workshop at Bethesda, Maryland, December 17–18, 2001. Radiat Res 159:812–834
31. Koana T, Takashima Y, Okada MO et al (2004) A threshold exists in the dose-response relationship for somatic mutation frequency induced by X irradiation of Drosophila. Radiat Res 161:391–396
32. Trotti A, Colevas AD, Setser A et al (2003) CTCAE v3.0: development of a comprehensive grading system for the adverse effects of cancer treatment. Semin Radiat Oncol 13:176–181
33. Coleman CN, Stone HB, Alexander GA et al (2003) Education and training for radiation scientists: radiation research program and American Society of Therapeutic Radiology and Oncology Workshop, Bethesda, Maryland, May 12–14, 2003. Radiat Res 160:729–737
34. Stone HB, Moulder JE, Coleman CN et al (2004) Models for evaluating agents intended for the prophylaxis, mitigation and treatment of radiation injuries. Report of an NCI Workshop, December 3–4, 2003. Radiat Res 162:711–728
35. Brizel DM, Wasserman TH, Henke M et al (2000) Phase III randomized trial of amifostine as a radioprotector in head and neck cancer. J Clin Oncol 18:3339–3345
36. Wasserman TH, Brizel DM (2001) The role of amifostine as a radioprotector. Oncology (Huntingt) 15:1349–1354; discussion 1357–1360
37. Hahn SM, Krishna MC, DeLuca AM et al (2000) Evaluation of the hydroxylamine Tempol-H as an in vivo radioprotector. Free Radic Biol Med 28:953–958
38. Metz JM, Smith D, Mick R et al (2004) A phase I study of topical Tempol for the prevention of alopecia induced by whole brain radiotherapy. Clin Cancer Res 10:6411–6417
39. Moulder JE, Fish BL, Cohen EP (2003) ACE inhibitors and AII receptor antagonists in the treatment and prevention of bone marrow transplant nephropathy. Curr Pharm Des 9:737–749
40. Moulder JE (2004) Post-irradiation approaches to treatment of radiation injuries in the context of radiological terrorism and radiation accidents: a review. Int J Radiat Biol 80 3–10
41. Delanian S, Lefaix JL (2002) Complete healing of severe osteoradionecrosis with treatment combining pentoxifylline, tocopherol and clodronate. Br J Radiol 75:467–469
42. Komarov PG, Komarova EA, Kondratov RV et al (1999) A chemical inhibitor of p53 that protects mice from the side effects of cancer therapy. Science 285:1733–1737
43. Komarova EA, Kondratov RV, Wang K et al (2004) Dual effect of p53 on radiation sensitivity in vivo: p53 promotes hematopoietic injury, but protects from gastro-intestinal syndrome in mice. Oncogene 23:3265–3271
44. Komarova EA, Christov K, Faerman AI et al (2000) Different impact of p53 and p21 on the radiation response of mouse tissues. Oncogene 19:3791–3798
45. Paris F, Fuks Z, Kang A et al (2001) Endothelial apoptosis as the primary lesion initiating intestinal radiation damage in mice. Science 293:293–297
46. Derynck R, Zhang YE (2003) Smad-dependent and Smad-independent pathways in TGF-beta family signalling. Nature 425:577–584
47. Nishioka A, Ogawa Y, Mima T et al (2004) Histopathologic amelioration of fibroproliferative change in rat irradiated lung using soluble transforming growth factor-beta (TGF-beta) receptor mediated by adenoviral vector. Int J Radiat Oncol Biol Phys 58:1235–1241
48. Rabbani ZN, Anscher MS, Zhang X et al (2003) Soluble TGFbeta type II receptor gene therapy ameliorates acute radiation-induced pulmonary injury in rats. Int J Radiat Oncol Biol Phys 57:563–572
49. Xavier S, Piek E, Fujii M et al (2004) Amelioration of radiation-induced fibrosis: inhibition of transforming growth factor-beta signaling by halofuginone. J Biol Chem 279:15167–15176
50. Pellmar TC, Rockwell S (2005) Priority list of research areas for radiological nuclear threat countermeasures. Radiat Res 163:115–123
51. Dorr W, Noack R, Spekl K et al (2001) Modification of oral mucositis by keratinocyte growth factor: single radiation exposure. Int J Radiat Biol 77:341–347
52. Waselenko JK, MacVittie TJ, Blakely WF et al (2004) Medical management of the acute radiation syndrome: recommendations of the Strategic National Stockpile Radiation Working Group. Ann Intern Med 140:1037–1051

Ionizing Radiation and the Endothelium – A Brief Review

LUIS FELIPE FAJARDO L-G

CONTENTS

3.1 Introduction 19
3.2 Physiology of Endothelial Cells 20
3.3 Effects of Radiation on Endothelial Cells 21
References 22

Presented at the LENT V WORKSHOP. Rochester, New York, May 19, 2004

Supported by: Department of Pathology, Stanford University, fund 1-HMZ-178 and Veterans Affairs Fund FAJ 0004

L. F. FAJARDO L-G, MD
Professor, Department of Pathology, Stanford University School of Medicine, and Veterans Affairs Medical Center, 3801 Miranda Avenue, Palo Alto, CA 94304, USA

Summary

Endothelial cells (EC) are the most radiosensitive among the fixed elements of the mesenchyme. Depending on dose, ionizing radiation can produce lethal or sublethal injury to EC. The latter may alter considerably the complex physiology of the endothelium. Some functions are inhibited or abolished: fibrinolysis, synthesis of various enzymes and cytokines, attachment of EC to the basal lamina, angiogenesis, etc.

Other functions are enhanced, including permeability, soluble coagulation, platelet adhesion, and aggregation. There is also upregulation of adhesion molecules for leukocytes. Endothelial cells are heterogeneous; accordingly, radiation effects vary in quality and severity from one site to another, and from one animal species to another.

3.1 Introduction

Blood vessels are important targets of radiation in normal and neoplastic mammalian tissues; in fact, many early and delayed radiation effects are mediated through vascular injury [1–3]. Endothelial cells (EC) are key elements of the vessel wall, present at all levels of the vascular tree, and their integrity is essential for vascular function [4]. This description summarizes in vivo and in vitro data indicating the role of EC in the pathologic processes produced by ionizing radiation.

3.2 Physiology of Endothelial Cells

A discussion of the radiation effects on endothelial cells should be preceded by some review of the complex physiology of the endothelium [4]. Aside from those activities common to all cells, certain specialized functions are characteristic of EC [4]:

- Coagulation: EC participate in the soluble coagulation system by producing both procoagulants (e.g. tissue factor and Factor V) and anticoagulants (e.g. plasminogen activators and thrombomodulin.). In addition EC regulate the adhesion and aggregation of platelets through von Willebrand Factor (vWill F), nitric oxide, etc.
- Permeability: transport of certain molecules across the EC cytoplasm.
- Inflammation and immune response: EC express multiple antigens, including MHCs I and II, and ABO. Several cytokines are produced in EC, such as IL1 and GM-CSF. Depending on activation state, lymphocytes, granulocytes, and macrophages adhere to specific EC receptors.
- Synthesis of stromal components: EC produce their own basement membrane (mainly collagens IV, V, and laminin), as well as various collagens for the surrounding tissue matrix.
- Vascular tone regulation: Through angiotensin converting enzyme and endothelin, EC contract smooth muscle while nitric oxide relaxes it.
- Angiogenesis: This, the formation of microvessels in the fully developed vertebrate, is the most dynamic function of the endothelium; it occurs in response to a large number of agonists and antagonists. It is either physiologic (e.g., in wound healing and cyclical endometrial growth) or pathologic (e.g., in neoplasia and many inflammatory diseases) [4, 5].

The above, and other endothelial cell functions, are regulated by numerous genes, many of which have been characterized [6]. EC vary greatly from tissue to tissue and from one animal species to another. This heterogeneity is evident morphologically, functionally, and in response to injury [4].

Figure 3.1 outlines diagrammatically the most important of the functions characteristic of EC (compare with Fig. 3.2).

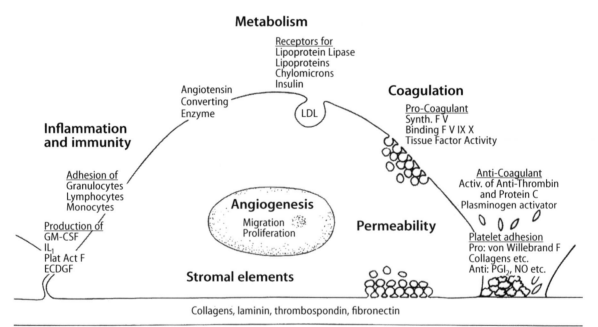

L. Fajardo

Fig. 3.1. A normal endothelial cell attached to its basal lamina (*bottom*), which is partially denuded on the right. The main functions described here are indicated in *bold uppercase letters*, with examples in *lowercase*. *ABO*, blood antigens; *ACE*, angiotensin converting enzyme; *GM-CSF*, granulocyte-monocyte colony stimulating factor; *LDL*, low density lipoproteins; *MHC I & II*, major histocompatibility complexes; *NO*, nitric oxide; *PGI$_2$*, prostacyclin. (Reproduced, with permission, from [17])

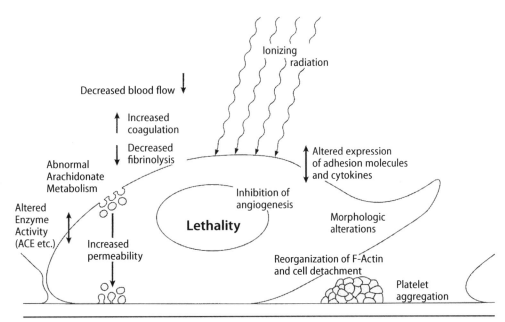

L. Fajardo

Fig. 3.2. General effects of radiation on endothelial cells. (Compare with Fig. 3.1.) This is a diagrammatical summary of the most important, lethal, and sublethal effects of ionizing radiation on endothelial cells. It combines in vitro and in vivo data and is based on multiple sources of information. (Reproduced, with permission, from [14])

3.3
Effects of Radiation on Endothelial Cells

The impact of ionizing radiation on the endothelium has been studied in vivo and in vitro, the latter using various EC lines, including human umbilical vein cells (HUVEC), bovine aortic cells (BAEC), or capillary EC (e.g., HDMEC). The doses varied between <1 Gy and as much as 60 Gy, with various fractionation schemes. For the in vitro studies, the doses were often 5 Gy or less. From a review of various in vitro experiments (too many to list here), it appears that radiation becomes lethal to endothelial cells when it reaches Do values in the order of 100–200 cGy in the clonogenic survival curves (higher values are required in vivo).

EC may undergo mitotic death or apoptosis, the latter through a pathway that probably involves the formation of ceramide [7].

Sublethal doses of radiation affect the morphology and various functions of EC.

Common morphologic changes include hypertrophy of EC associated with re-organization of F-actin filaments, and detachment from the basement membrane [8–11]. The in vivo changes include vascular constrictions, thromboses, and rupture of microvascular walls with resulting hypoperfusion [9]. Most studies show an increase in permeability for various molecules [12, 13] (however, serotonin transport is decreased [9]). There is hypercoagulation, and platelet aggregation due to enhanced release of vWill F, causing an increased tendency to thrombosis [14]. In addition, ineffective fibrinolysis results from a decrease in plasminogen activators [13]. The eicosanoid metabolism is altered, with early decrease and late increase in PGI-2 [13]. There is enhanced chemoattraction for leukocytes and upregulation of adhesion molecules (e.g., ELAM-1) [15]. EC show decrease in endothelial enzyme activity (e.g., angiotensin converting enzyme, alkaline phosphatase) [13]. Radiation inhibits angiogenesis [5]: The magnitude of this effect depends in part on the sequence of angiogenic stimulus vs radiation. Various data suggest that the inhibition of angiogenesis is greater when the radiation exposure occurs prior to the angiogenic stimulus instead of following it [2, 5]. This information may be important when designing the sequence of radiation therapy vs surgery (the angiogenic stimulus).

Like other normal cells, EC have some innate protection from ionizing radiation. For instance, glutathione and superoxide dismutase provide some defense of EC from reactive oxygen species (e.g., hydroxyl radical and superoxide respectively) [16]. Nevertheless it appears that endothelial cells are the most radiosensitive elements in the vessel wall [8]. They may even be the most sensitive among the fixed cells of the mesenchyme. Many of the studies suggest that EC are more radioresponsive in vitro than in vivo [7]. Sublethal endothelial radiation injury not only contributes to the very early, acute effects, but also accounts for many of the delayed effects, such as stromal fibrinous exudate and ischemia [14].

Several of the above described deleterious effects of radiation on the EC can be ameliorated or even abrogated by pharmacologic modifiers [13]. However, as far as we know, there is no single compound that prevents all of these effects in the endothelium.

Vascular injury is a price to be paid for the successes of cancer radiotherapy.

References

1. Fajardo LF, Berthrong M (1988) Vascular lesions following radiation. Pathology Annual 23:297–330
2. Hopewell JW (1983) Radiation effects on vascular tissue. In: Potten CS, Hendry JH (eds) Cytotoxic insult to tissue. Churchill Livingstone, Edinburgh, pp 228–257
3. Reinhold HS, Hopewell JW (1980) Late changes in the architecture of blood vessels of the rat brain after irradiation. Br J Radiol 53:693–696
4. Fajardo LF (1989) The complexity of endothelial cells. A review. Am J Clin Path 92:241–250
5. Prionas SD, Kowalski J, Fajardo LF et al (1990) Effects of x-irradiation on angiogenesis. Radiat Res 124:43–49
6. Grove AD, Prabhu VV, Young BL et al (2002) Both protein activation and gene expression are involved in early vascular tube formation in vitro. Clin Cancer Res 8:3019–3026
7. Haimovitz-Friedman A, Fuks Z (1998) Signaling in the radiation response of endothelial cells. In: Rubin DB (ed) The radiation biology of the vascular endothelium. CRC Press, Boca Raton, pp 101–127
8. Johnson LK, Longenecker JP, Fajardo LF (1982) Differential radiation response of cultured endothelial cells and smooth myocytes. Anal Quant Cytol 4:188–198
9. Kwock L, Blackstock AW Friedman M (1998) Effect of ionizing radiation on endothelial cell plasma membrane processes. In: Rubin DB (ed) The radiation biology of the vascular endothelium. CRC Press, Boca Raton, pp 129–145
10. Onoda JM, Kantak SS, Diglio CA (1998) Extracellular matrix regulates endothelial cell morphology, receptor expression, and response to low dose radiation. In: Rubin DB (ed) The radiation biology of the vascular endothelium. CRC Press, Boca Raton, pp 161–183
11. Rosen EM, Goldberg ID (1998) Protein synthesis in irradiated endothelial cells. In: Rubin DB (ed) The radiation biology of the vascular endothelium. CRC Press, Boca Raton, pp 95–100
12. Graham MM, Peterson LM (1998) Functional measures of endothelial integrity and pharmacologic modifications of radiation injury. In: Rubin DB (ed) The radiation biology of the vascular endothelium. CRC Press, Boca Raton, pp 39–64
13. Ward DC, Molteni JV, Ts'ao Ch (1998) Endothelial-oriented strategies to spare normal tissues. In: Rubin DB (ed) The radiation biology of the vascular endothelium. CRC Press, Boca Raton, pp 185–208
14. Fajardo LF (1998) The endothelial cell is a unique target of radiation: an overview. In: Rubin DB (ed) The radiation biology of the vascular endothelium. CRC Press, Boca Raton, pp 1–12
15. Murray JC (1998) Inflammatory cytokines, radiation and endothelial gene products: a common role for reactive oxygen intermediates. In: Rubin DB (ed) The radiation biology of the vascular endothelium. CRC Press, Boca Raton, pp 147–160
16. Rubin DFB, Drab EA, Blazek ER (1998) Antioxidant defenses and the irradiated endothelium. In: Rubin DB (ed) The radiation biology of the vascular endothelium. CRC Press, Boca Raton, pp 65–89
17. Fajardo LF (1989) The unique physiology of endothelial cells and its implications in radiobiology. Front Radiat Ther Oncol 23:96–112

Inflammation and Cell Adhesion Molecules are Involved in Radiation-Induced Lung Injury

Christopher D. Willey and Dennis E. Hallahan

CONTENTS

4.1 Introduction 23
4.2 Radiation-Induced Lung Injury 24
4.2.2 Transcriptional Regulation of Inflammatory Mediators 24
4.2.3 Inflammation and Fibrosis 25
4.3 Inhibitors of Radiation-Induced Inflammation 27
4.4 Future Goals 29
References 29

Summary

Radiation therapy is an effective means of killing tumor cells, although this effectiveness is tempered by limitations of the normal tissue to the adverse effects of radiation. An excellent example of this is radiation treatment for thoracic tumors, in particular, lung cancers. Despite advances in the technical delivery of radiation by three-dimensional (3D) planning via computed tomography (CT), radiation-induced injury to normal lung tissue still occurs in a large proportion of treated patients. The primary endpoints for radiation-induced pulmonary toxicity include early onset pneumonitis and late onset fibrosis. A significant amount of research has produced some insight into the mechanism(s) behind this injury. This knowledge has provided potential targets for drug development that could improve the therapeutic ratio for radiation by reducing both early and late toxicity. In this article, we review and update the pathologic mechanisms underlying radiation-induced lung injury as well as potential treatments, with particular interest in cell adhesion molecules and inflammation.

4.1 Introduction

The ability to successfully treat cancer using radiation therapy is as dependent upon normal tissue tolerance as it is upon tumor cell kill. Indeed, radiation treatment to tumors that lie within delicate organs poses a great challenge to the radiation oncologist. One of the most pertinent examples is that of thoracic tumors which account for more than 400,000 patients per year in the US [1]. Radiation treatment is used in the majority of these patients and, due to the inherent sensitivity of the lungs, radiation-induced injury limits the effective treatment. Indeed, 5%–15% of patients will develop pneumonitis and an even larger percentage will develop evidence of fibrosis [2]. Numerous risk factors have been implicated in the development of radiation-induced lung injury; these include: certain mutations in chromosomes 1, 17, and 18, chemotherapy exposure, large radiation volume, high dose rate, high dose, and positive smoking status [2–5]. Several studies have elucidated the impact of the dosimetric delivery of radiation, as well as the radiobiological and molecular biological determinants of radiation-induced injury to the lungs [6]. Reviews of technical aspects in the development of radiation pneumonitis have been presented elsewhere [7, 8]. The content of this review will be focused on the biology of tissue injury, in particular, the inflammatory mediators involved.

C. D. Willey, MD, PhD
D. E. Hallahan, MD
Department of Radiation Oncology, The Vanderbilt Ingram Cancer Center, Vanderbilt University Medical Center, Nashville, TN 37232, USA

4.2
Radiation-Induced Lung Injury

There are two general categories of radiation-induced lung injury that can be distinguished somewhat temporally, acute phase pneumonitis and late phase fibrosis. Radiation pneumonitis typically occurs within the first 6 months of treatment, whereas lung fibrosis occurs months to years after treatment [1, 3]. Pneumonitis presents with symptoms reminiscent of pneumonia with low-grade fever, cough, and dyspnea. On the other hand, fibrosis presents with a more chronic picture, with dyspnea and cyanosis. Based on current scientific knowledge, less is known about the pathophysiology of fibrosis. Pneumonitis, on the other hand, has attracted considerable interest such that a great deal is known about the signaling involved in this acute radiation injury process. However, we are beginning to see that these two processes are probably linked despite the differences that are seen clinically and histologically [3, 7].

It is generally accepted that the target cells of radiation injury in the lung are the type II pneumocytes and vascular endothelium. In response to toxic stresses, type I pneumocytes seem to be damaged relatively easily, while the type II pneumocytes proliferate in response to injury [7, 9, 10]. Eventually, these type II pneumocytes repopulate the alveolar surface and some convert to type I pneumocytes, since the type I cannot self-renew [2]. Many believe that it is the inhibition of type II pneumocytes that leads to radiation-induced fibrosis. However, it is becoming increasingly clear that inflammatory cells that are recruited contribute to this process by releasing pro-inflammatory cytokines. Rubin et al. was probably the first group to emphasize this idea of signal transduction of cytokines or the "cascade of cytokines" [11]. Their studies of rabbit lungs identified differences between irradiated and normal macrophages in terms of transforming growth factor (TGF) production, with the former being enhanced [12]. These studies have paved the way for further investigation into the role of these inflammatory cells. As such, we now know that pulmonary macrophages and lymphocytes triggered from the radiation not only affect the irradiated area, but also spread to surrounding tissue. This likely explains why the pneumonitis volume can exceed the treated volume [9, 13].

When analyzed microscopically, it is clear that the cellular damage from radiation becomes evident within hours even though the end products of pneumonitis and fibrosis do not occur for many weeks to months [7]. Almost immediately after radiation insult, type II pneumocytes have a visible decrease in their lamellar bodies while they release surfactant into the alveolar space. Over the next several hours, damage to the endothelium results in increased permeability that is apparent as perivascular edema. Within weeks, a great deal of proliferation produces changes in the alveolar walls that begin to fill with numerous cell types, including fibroblasts that lay down collagen fibrils [7, 14]. Ultimately, the capillaries are destroyed by the fibrotic process, while additional type II pneumocytes and vascular smooth muscle cells fill the septae [7]. Eventually, capillaries may regenerate, but chronic fibrosis is certainly a possible adverse outcome from radiation damage, particularly if the type II pneumocytes are inhibited [9].

4.2.2
Transcriptional Regulation of Inflammatory Mediators

The potential signal transduction pathways that are activated by radiation are numerous, including apoptotic pathways via sphingomyelin and ceramide [15, 16], as well as direct genetic damage to the cell [17]. However, an interesting set of stress response genes are activated within the irradiated cells, many of which are involved in the inflammatory process. Indeed, upregulation of NF-κB, as well as the early response genes, namely c-abl, c-fos, c-jun, and egr-1, activate the cells to produce cytokines that amplify the inflammatory process [1–3, 7]. Specifically, we have shown that NF-κB can be activated via reactive oxygen species generated from radiation. This process leads to the induction of a pro-inflammatory cascade including TNFα [18, 19]. In addition, it has become well known that growth factors are also released, particularly TGF-β. TGF-β has been implicated in the actual lung fibrosis that occurs following radiation insult. In fact, several groups have studied TGF-β levels within patients receiving radiation and have suggested that it is a marker for radiation pneumonitis [20–26].

Microarray analysis of irradiated endothelial cells has allowed for the identification of other potential mediators involved in the inflammatory process. We have identified two radiation-inducible cell adhesion molecules that appear to be key players in the development of radiation pneumonitis. These two molecules are intercellular adhesion molecule 1

(ICAM-1) and E-selectin [27]. Interestingly, knock-out studies have shown that E-selectin deletion is insufficient to modify radiation pneumonitis due to redundancy with P-selectin [28]. ICAM-1, on the other hand, has proven to be even more interesting, as shown in Fig. 4.1. The production of ICAM-1 increases substantially immediately following irradiation of mouse lung (four-fold within 2 days of treatment). However, it is not until day 28 post-irradiation that ICAM-1 production peaks (Fig. 4.1). This late increase in ICAM-1 is reflective of the delayed nature of radiation fibrosis and pneumonitis. It is felt that the ICAM-I production provides a place of attachment for leukocytes that are recruited to the vicinity that essentially provides a positive feedback loop.

It should be noted that studies using a pig model have suggested less of a role for ICAM-1. Kasper et al. have published data that shows a loss of ICAM-1 expression during the inflammatory phase and purport that ICAM-1 is not expressed by alveolar epithelial cells that are within fibrotic lesions [29]. Despite this alternative viewpoint, our extensive studies using both ICAM-1 inhibitors and ICAM-1 knockout mice [30, 31] show that ICAM-1 expression and function are critical players in radiation injury. In addition, data from other organs support our hypothesis of ICAM-I activation during radiation injury. Specifically, ICAM-I up-regulation has been demonstrated to have a dose response to radiation at the blood–brain barrier [32], within irradiation rat colonic tissue [33], as well as in human head and neck cancer patients [34].

Other laboratories have identified tissue hypoxia as playing a central role in generating the inflammatory process. Vujaskovic et al. have shown that radiation can induce hypoxia that contributes to late normal tissue injury. They contend that the hypoxia following radiation results in progressive tissue damage that perpetuates the production of reactive oxygen species (ROS) that also helps produce cytokines. They identified by immunohistochemistry the induction of VEGF, TGF-β, and CD-31 in the late responding rat lung tissue [35]. Moreover, Epperly et al. have provided evidence showing a connection between ROS and the adhesion molecules ICAM-I and VCAM-I. They showed that the addition of the ROS scavenger, manganese superoxide dismutase, could attenuate the expression of these molecules [36]. These studies add further support to an inflammatory-based mechanism of radiation-induced lung injury.

4.2.3 Inflammation and Fibrosis

Current models of radiation pneumonitis tend to separate the inflammatory process from the fibrosis process. It is suggested that the radiation triggers cells to release inflammatory cytokines such as TNF-α, IL-1, IL-6, and various other chemokines that help recruit macrophages and lymphocytes to the damaged area, which further enhances the production of those cytokines [3, 37]. Eventually, the interplay between the alveolar epithelium, the endothelium, recruited macrophages and lymphocytes, as well as the fibroblasts and leukocytes triggers the production of the fibrotic cytokines, namely basic fibroblast growth factor (bFGF), TGF-β, and platelet-derived growth factor (PDGF) [37, 38]. The complex interaction among these chemical signalers leads to fibroblast proliferation and collagen formation: in essence, the fibrosis. Indeed, foci of inflammation within areas of irradiated lung coincide with fibrotic sites [39]. This connection between inflammation and the fibrosis that leads to lung injury provides some interesting targets for therapy that may abrogate the process (Table 4.1).

Studies by our lab have demonstrated that ICAM-1 may be a critical player not only in the development of pneumonitis but also in the production of pulmonary fibrosis in response to radiation. Hallahan et al. have demonstrated that genetic targeting of

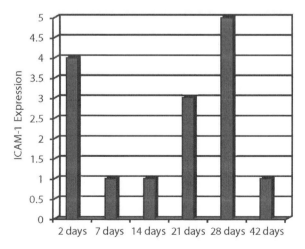

Fig. 4.1. Time course of ICAM-1 expression in irradiated mouse lung. The fold-increase in ICAM-1 expression normalized to pre-irradiation levels is plotted against the elapsed time in days following irradiation with 14 Gy

Table 4.1. Table of implicated inflammatory regulators [1, 7, 37]

Proposed inflammatory regulators		
PDGF	L-selectin	Prostacyclin
bFGF	E-selectin	Plasminogen activator
MCP-1	RANTES	TNF-α
IL-1α	Angiotensin converting enzyme (ACE)	VEGF
IL-6	MIP-1α, -1β, and -2	Lymphotactin
TGF-β	Interferon inducible protein-10 (IP-10)	Eotaxin

ICAM-1 both attenuates the inflammatory response to radiation within the lungs of mice and prevents the fibrosis from occurring months after the radiation [31]. ICAM-1 null mice are severely limited in their ability to recruit inflammatory cells following radiation treatment. We show in Figure 4.2 that the mean number of LCA-positive cells is reduced below untreated control levels when ICAM-1 −/− mice are compared with wild type. Interestingly, there is a reduction in alveolar septal wall thickness (Fig. 4.3), amount of collagen type III deposition (Fig. 4.4), and pulmonary stiffness that occurs 6–9 months after ICAM-1 −/− are treated with radiation. Indeed, we have shown that the incidence of respiratory distress is lower in ICAM-1 −/− mice 12 months post-irradiation (Fig. 4.5), demonstrating that lung injury can be attenuated by blocking the ICAM-1 pathway.

One of the main upstream regulators of ICAM and E-selectin is NF-κB. This transcription factor is normally sequestered within the cytoplasm by its inhibitor, IκB. However, when IκB is phosphorylated, NF-κB becomes released and translocates into the nucleus in order to modulate gene expression. When the cis regulatory element of NF-κB is deleted, ICAM and E-selectin promoters cannot be induced [40]. There are several kinases that can activate the NF-κB pathway, but the phosphatidylinositol-3 kinase (PI3K)/Akt pathway is a likely candidate for radiation-induced activation. We have clearly demonstrated that radiation induces the activation of PI3K, which subsequently phosphorylates and activates Akt in a dose-dependent manner [41–43]. Once stimulated, Akt can activate transcription factors such as NF-κB, Forkhead, and CREB, but also downregulate pro-apoptotic proteins such as Bad and Caspase-9 [44–46]. PI3K, thus, has become an attractive target for inhibition in the

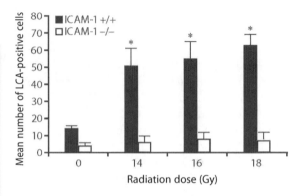

Fig. 4.2. Attenuated radiation-induced pulmonary inflammation in ICAM-1 −/− mice. Groups of 10 ICAM-1 −/− and ICAM-1 +/+ mice were irradiated at the doses indicated. At 5 weeks post-irradiation, the animals were sacrificed, and lungs were prepared for histologic staining for leukocyte-common antigen (LCA). LCA positive cells were counted for both the ICAM-1 −/− and ICAM-1 +/+ mice. The *asterisk* indicates statistical significance. (Reprinted from [31] with permission of Oxford University Press)

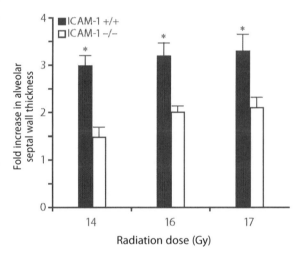

Fig. 4.3. Alveolar wall thickness as a measure of lung fibrosis in ICAM-1 −/− mice. Groups of 10 ICAM-1 −/− and ICAM-1 +/+ mice were irradiated at the doses indicated. Those animals that survived for 18 months post-irradiation were sacrificed, and lungs were prepared for sectioning. Alveolar septal wall thickness was measured for five sections in each group. Fold increase in wall thickness normalized to non-irradiated mice is shown. *Asterisk* indicates statistical significance. (Reprinted from [31] with permission of Oxford University Press)

context of radiation resistance. However, PI3K inhibition can also be applied to the prevention and treatment of radiation-induced pneumonitis, as described below.

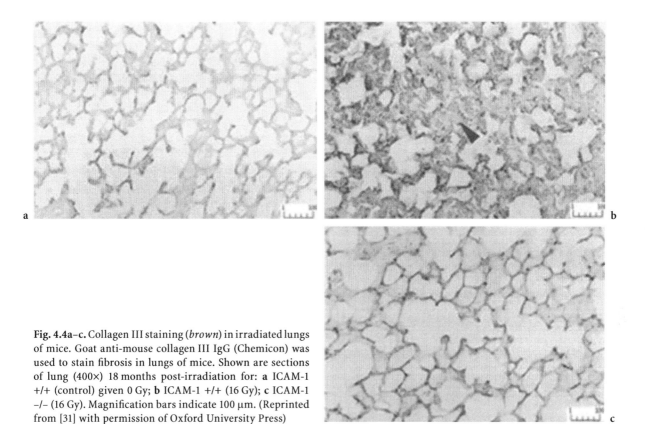

Fig. 4.4a–c. Collagen III staining (*brown*) in irradiated lungs of mice. Goat anti-mouse collagen III IgG (Chemicon) was used to stain fibrosis in lungs of mice. Shown are sections of lung (400×) 18 months post-irradiation for: **a** ICAM-1 +/+ (control) given 0 Gy; **b** ICAM-1 +/+ (16 Gy); **c** ICAM-1 –/– (16 Gy). Magnification bars indicate 100 μm. (Reprinted from [31] with permission of Oxford University Press)

Fig. 4.5. Percentage of mice showing respiratory distress after thoracic irradiation. Groups of 10 ICAM-1 –/– and ICAM-1 +/+ mice were irradiated at the doses indicated. Those animals were then observed for the onset of respiratory distress over the course of 18 months post-irradiation. This data is presented as percentage of mice in each group that displayed respiratory distress. *Asterisk* indicates $P=0.0036$ (general linear model). (Reprinted from [31] with permission of Oxford University Press)

4.3
Inhibitors of Radiation-Induced Inflammation

Because of the intimate connection between inflammation and fibrosis it is possible that targeting of inflammatory mediators might provide attenuation of the fibrotic process and reduce the possibility of radiation pneumonitis. As described above, ICAM-1 is a protein that is clearly involved in radiation-induced pulmonary injury and fibrosis in the mouse model. Therefore, targeting the upstream regulator, PI3K, can possibly reverse and/or prevent this ICAM-1-mediated fibrosis. Several isoform-specific inhibitors of PI3K have been developed, including one that targets the p110δ isoform known to be activated within the endothelium [42]. By treating endothelial cells with this compound, the induction of ICAM-1 can be eliminated following radiation, as shown in Figure. 4.6.

Several promising agents are being investigated to target various portions of the inflammation cascade, as well as angiogenic and fibrinogenic cascades. Table 4.2 lists several of these, including statins, thalidomide, and amifostine. The pathways summary in Figure 4.7 shows our working model for radiation-induced lung injury. Clearly, there are several places that these drugs could impact signal transduction.

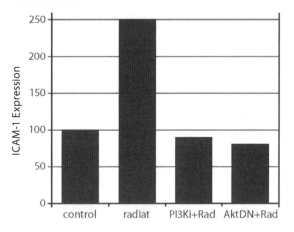

Fig. 4.6. PI3K/Akt inhibition and ICAM-1 expression in endothelium. Endothelium was treated with either mock irradiation (control) or 3 Gy irradiation either alone (radiat), with 200 nM PI3K inhibitor pre-treatment (PI3Ki + Rad), or adenoviral dominant negative Akt (AktDN + Rad). Percent ICAM-1 expression over the control is shown

Table 4.2. Potential therapeutics for radiation induced lung injury [1, 7]

Agent	Proposed mechanism
Pentoxifylline	Anti-fibrotic
Vitamin E	ROS scavenger
Chinese herb 764-1	Surfactant inhibitor
Corticosteroids	Anti-inflammatory
Captopril	IL-2 stimulation, ROS scavenger, Anti-TGF-β
Amifostine (WR-2721)	ROS scavenger
Super oxide dismutase	ROS scavenger
Statins	Chemokine inhibition
Keratinocyte growth factor (KGF)	Anti-apoptosis; mucosal protectant
Fibroblast growth factor 4 (FGF-4)	Anti-apoptosis
Thalidomide	Anti-angiogenic and cytokine inhibitor
Halofuginone	Anti-fibrotic/anti-TGF-β
IC489666	PI3K inhibitor

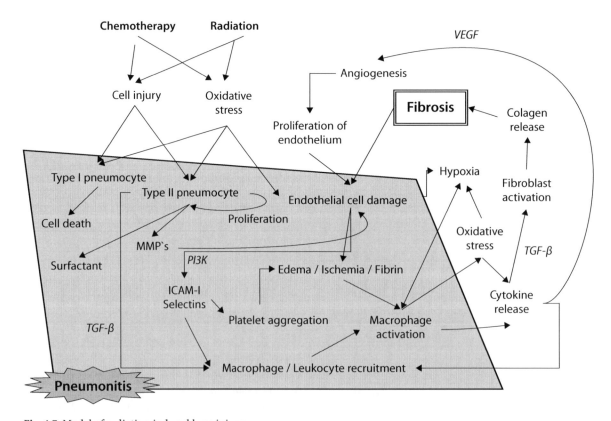

Fig. 4.7. Model of radiation-induced lung injury

4.4
Future Goals

Our studies involving ICAM-1 and radiation have provided a model for testing potential therapeutics in a preclinical setting. However, the translation to the clinic requires additional work in our preclinical model. Our published studies have involved the use of radiation alone as the means of inducing lung injury. However, it is rare that radiation is used as a single modality for lung cancer in clinical practice. More likely, chemotherapy is employed as a combined modality approach that introduces additional variables for the modeling of clinical radiation pneumonitis within the mouse model. Our studies need to be extended to include platinum-based chemotherapy concurrent with radiation treatment to further characterize the impact of ICAM-1 in terms of lung injury.

As molecular and cellular biology techniques have advanced, so too has our understanding of the pathophysiology of radiation-induced lung injury. Despite our scientific advances, many questions remain unanswered.

Acknowledgements

The authors wish to acknowledge Ross Summer for his helpful insights as a pulmonologist.

References

1. Stone HB, Moulder JE, Coleman CN et al (2004) Models for evaluating agents intended for the prophylaxis, mitigation and treatment of radiation injuries report of an NCI Workshop, December 3–4, 2003. Radiation Research 162:711–728
2. Abid SH, Malhotra V, Perry MC (2001) Radiation-induced and chemotherapy-induced pulmonary injury. Curr Opin Oncol 13:242–248
3. Marks LB, Yu X, Vujaskovic Z et al (2003) Radiation-induced lung injury. Semin Radiat Oncol 13:333–345
4. Monson JM, Stark P, Reilly JJ et al (1998) Clinical radiation pneumonitis and radiographic changes after thoracic radiation therapy for lung carcinoma. Cancer 82:842–850
5. Rancati T, Ceresoli GL, Gagliardi G et al (2003) Factors predicting radiation pneumonitis in lung cancer patients: a retrospective study. Radiother Oncol 67:275–283
6. Claude L, Perol D, Ginestet C et al (2004) A prospective study on radiation pneumonitis following conformal radiation therapy in non-small-cell lung cancer: clinical and dosimetric factors analysis. Radiother Oncol 71:175–181
7. Movsas B, Raffin TA, Epstein AH et al (1997) Pulmonary radiation injury. Chest 111:1061–1076
8. Rodrigues G, Lock M, D'Souza D et al (2004) Prediction of radiation pneumonitis by dose – volume histogram parameters in lung cancer – a systematic review. Radiother Oncol 71:127–138
9. Trott KR, Herrmann T, Kasper M (2004) Target cells in radiation pneumopathy. Int J Radiat Oncol Biol Phys 58:463–469
10. Osterreicher J, Pejchal J, Skopek J et al (2004) Role of type II pneumocytes in pathogenesis of radiation pneumonitis: dose response of radiation-induced lung changes in the transient high vascular permeability period. Exp Toxicol Pathol 56:181–187
11. Rubin P, Johnston CJ, Williams JP et al (1995) A perpetual cascade of cytokines postirradiation leads to pulmonary fibrosis. Int J Radiat Oncol Biol Phys 33:99–109
12. Rubin P, Finkelstein J, Shapiro D (1992) Molecular biology mechanisms in the radiation induction of pulmonary injury syndromes: interrelationship between the alveolar macrophage and the septal fibroblast. Int J Radiat Oncol Biol Phys 24:93–101
13. Roberts CM, Foulcher E, Zaunders JJ et al (1993) Radiation pneumonitis: a possible lymphocyte-mediated hypersensitivity reaction. Ann Intern Med 118:696–700
14. Ward HE, Kemsley L, Davies L et al (1993) The pulmonary response to sublethal thoracic irradiation in the rat. Radiat Res 136:15–21
15. Vit JP, Rosselli F (2003) Role of the ceramide-signaling pathways in ionizing radiation-induced apoptosis. Oncogene 22:8645–8652
16. Kolesnick R, Fuks Z (2003) Radiation and ceramide-induced apoptosis. Oncogene 22:5897–5906
17. Gross NJ (1981) The pathogenesis of radiation-induced lung damage. Lung 159:115–125
18. Hallahan DE, Spriggs DR, Beckett MA et al (1989) Increased tumor necrosis factor alpha mRNA after cellular exposure to ionizing radiation. Proc Natl Acad Sci USA 86:10104–10107
19. Hallahan DE, Virudachalam S, Kuchibhotla J et al (1994) Membrane-derived second messenger regulates X-ray-mediated tumor necrosis factor alpha gene induction. Proc Natl Acad Sci USA 91:4897–4901
20. Chen Y, Williams J, Ding I et al (2002) Radiation pneumonitis and early circulatory cytokine markers. Semin Radiat Oncol 12:26–33
21. Anscher MS, Peters WP, Reisenbichler H et al (1993) Transforming growth factor beta as a predictor of liver and lung fibrosis after autologous bone marrow transplantation for advanced breast cancer. N Engl J Med 328:1592–1598
22. Anscher MS, Kong FM, Marks LB et al (1997) Changes in plasma transforming growth factor beta during radiotherapy and the risk of symptomatic radiation-induced pneumonitis. Int J Radiat Oncol Biol Phys 37:253–258
23. Anscher MS, Murase T, Prescott DM et al (1994) Changes in plasma TGF beta levels during pulmonary radiotherapy as a predictor of the risk of developing radiation pneumonitis. Int J Radiat Oncol Biol Phys 30:671–676
24. Novakova-Jiresova A, Van Gameren MM, Coppes RP et al (2004) Transforming growth factor-beta plasma dy-

namics and post-irradiation lung injury in lung cancer patients. Radiother Oncol 71:183–189
25. De Jaeger K, Seppenwoolde Y, Kampinga HH et al (2004) Significance of plasma transforming growth factor-beta levels in radiotherapy for non-small-cell lung cancer. Int J Radiat Oncol Biol Phys 58:1378–1387
26. Barthelemy-Brichant N, Bosquee L, Cataldo D et al (2004) Increased IL-6 and TGF-beta1 concentrations in bronchoalveolar lavage fluid associated with thoracic radiotherapy. Int J Radiat Oncol Biol Phys 58:758–767
27. Hallahan DE, Virudachalam S (1997) Ionizing radiation mediates expression of cell adhesion molecules in distinct histological patterns within the lung. Cancer Res 57:2096–2099
28. Epperly MW, Guo H, Shields D et al (2004) Correlation of ionizing irradiation-induced late pulmonary fibrosis with long-term bone marrow culture fibroblast progenitor cell biology in mice homozygous deletion recombinant negative for endothelial cell adhesion molecules. In Vivo 18:1–14
29. Kasper M, Koslowski R, Luther T et al (1995) Immunohistochemical evidence for loss of ICAM-1 by alveolar epithelial cells in pulmonary fibrosis. Histochem Cell Biol 104:397–405
30. Hallahan DE, Virudachalam S (1997) Intercellular adhesion molecule 1 knockout abrogates radiation induced pulmonary inflammation. Proc Natl Acad Sci USA 94:6432–6437
31. Hallahan DE, Geng L, Shyr Y (2002) Effects of intercellular adhesion molecule 1 (ICAM-1) null mutation on radiation-induced pulmonary fibrosis and respiratory insufficiency in mice. J Natl Cancer Inst 94:733–741
32. Nordal RA, Wong CS (2004) Intercellular adhesion molecule-1 and blood-spinal cord barrier disruption in central nervous system radiation injury. J Neuropathol Exp Neurol 63:474–483
33. Ikeda Y, Ito M, Matsuu M et al (2000) Expression of ICAM-1 and acute inflammatory cell infiltration in the early phase of radiation colitis in rats. J Radiat Res (Tokyo) 41:279–291
34. Handschel J, Prott FJ, Sunderkotter C et al (1999) Irradiation induces increase of adhesion molecules and accumulation of beta2-integrin-expressing cells in humans. Int J Radiat Oncol Biol Phys 45:475–481
35. Vujaskovic Z, Anscher MS, Feng QF et al (2001) Radiation-induced hypoxia may perpetuate late normal tissue injury. Int J Radiat Oncol Biol Phys 50:851–855
36. Epperly MW, Sikora CA, DeFilippi SJ et al (2002) Pulmonary irradiation-induced expression of VCAM-I and ICAM-I is decreased by manganese superoxide dismutase-plasmid/liposome (MnSOD-PL) gene therapy. Biol Blood Marrow Transplant 8:175–187
37. Chen Y, Okunieff P, Ahrendt SA (2003) Translational research in lung cancer. Semin Surg Oncol 21:205–219
38. Thornton SC, Walsh BJ, Bennett S et al (1996) Both in vitro and in vivo irradiation are associated with induction of macrophage-derived fibroblast growth factors. Clin Exp Immunol 103:67–73
39. Franko AJ, Sharplin J, Ghahary A et al (1997) Immunohistochemical localization of transforming growth factor beta and tumor necrosis factor alpha in the lungs of fibrosis-prone and «non-fibrosing» mice during the latent period and early phase after irradiation. Radiat Res 147:245–256
40. Hallahan DE, Virudachalam S, Kuchibhotla J (1998) Nuclear factor kappaB dominant negative genetic constructs inhibit X-ray induction of cell adhesion molecules in the vascular endothelium. Cancer Res 58:5484–5488
41. Edwards E, Geng L, Tan J et al (2002) Phosphatidylinositol 3-kinase/Akt signaling in the response of vascular endothelium to ionizing radiation. Cancer Res 62:4671–4677
42. Geng L, Tan J, Himmelfarb E et al (2004) A specific antagonist of the p110delta catalytic component of phosphatidylinositol 3'-kinase, IC486068, enhances radiation-induced tumor vascular destruction. Cancer Res 64:4893–4899
43. Tan J, Hallahan DE (2003) Growth factor-independent activation of protein kinase B contributes to the inherent resistance of vascular endothelium to radiation-induced apoptotic response. Cancer Res 63:7663–7667
44. Kim D, Dan HC, Park S et al (2005) AKT/PKB signaling mechanisms in cancer and chemoresistance. Front Biosci 10:975–984
45. Parsa AT, Holland EC (2004) Cooperative translational control of gene expression by Ras and Akt in cancer. Trends Mol Med 10:607–613
46. Thompson JE, Thompson CB (2004) Putting the rap on Akt. J Clin Oncol 22:4217–4226

Volume Effects in Radiation Damage to Rat Lung

Richard P. Hill, Mohammed A. Khan, Aimee R. Langan, Ivan W.T. Yeung, and Jake Van Dyk

CONTENTS

5.1 Introduction 32
5.2 Materials and Methods 32
5.3 Results 33
5.4 Discussion 35
References 36

Paper presented at the Late Effects of Normal Tissue-V Workshop
at
University of Rochester School of Medicine and Department of Radiation Oncology, University of Rochester Medical Center, Rochester, New York

R. P. Hill, PhD
A. R. Langan, MD
Research Division, Ontario Cancer Institute, Princess Margaret Hospital, University Health Network, Departments of Medical Biophysics and Radiation Oncology, University of Toronto, 610 University Ave., Toronto, Ontario M5G 2M9, Canada
M. A. Khan, MD
Research Division, Ontario Cancer Institute, Princess Margaret Hospital, University Health Network, 610 University Ave., Toronto, Ontario M5G 2M9, Canada
I. W. T. Yeung, MD
Radiation Medicine Department, Princess Margaret Hospital, University Health Network, 610 University Ave., Toronto, Ontario M5G 2M9, Canada
J. Van Dyk, MD
Radiation Treatment Program, London Regional Cancer Program, London Health Sciences Centre, 790 Commissioners Road, London, Ontario, N6A 4L6, Canada

Summary

Purpose: Previously we have reported that DNA damage (micronuclei) observed in cells (fibroblasts) derived from the rat lung following irradiation is present in shielded regions of the lung apex following irradiation of the lung base. The present studies extend these observations to examine the effect of partial-volume irradiation of the lung base.

Methods and materials: The lungs of Sprague-Dawley rats were locally irradiated with 10 Gy ^{60}Co γ-rays; 18 h later the lungs were removed and divided into different quadrants before the preparation of a cell suspension. DNA damage was quantified in the lung cells using a micronucleus assay.

Results: Following irradiation of the whole rat lung, higher levels (10%–15%) of DNA damage were observed in the lung base vs. the lung apex and in the left lung vs. the right lung. Similar left–right differences were observed following irradiation of the lung base (70% of lung volume) both in-field and out-of-field in the shielded regions of the lung apex. Partial volume irradiation of the left or right lung base demonstrated that the extent of DNA damage in the shielded left or right apex was ipsilateral and dependent on the volume of the lung base irradiated.

Conclusions: Significant differences in early DNA damage are observed in different regions of the rat lung both in and out of the radiation field. The extent of damage is highly dependent on the volume and region of the lung that is irradiated.

5.1
Introduction

The effect of irradiating different volumes of the lung is complex and has been reported to depend on both the volume and region of the lung irradiated. In mice, irradiation of a volume in the apex of the lung caused less functional deficit than irradiation of a similar volume in the base of the lung [1, 2]. We have reported similar volume effects in rats using an early endpoint involving the examination of DNA damage (micronucleus formation) in cells (fibroblasts) derived from different irradiated regions of the lung [3, 4]. In these studies we found that the left lung demonstrated more DNA damage than the right lung following whole lung irradiation. Weigman et al. [5] also observed difference in lung response following irradiation of different regions of rat lung (always 50% of the volume); they observed changes in breathing rate only following irradiation of the left lung. CT density changes were most pronounced following irradiation of the left lung and the mediastinum. The reasons for these regional differences in response remain unclear but it has been postulated that they are due either to different numbers of functional sub-units in the base and apex of the lung [6] or to the induction of indirect effects associated with cytokine production induced by the irradiation [4]. Studies in pig lung, using both imaging and functional (breathing rate) endpoints, also observed greater functional effects after irradiating a greater volume of lung, but did not report regional differences [7, 8].

A surprising aspect of the regional effects observed by ourselves [4] was that DNA damage is found in cells from regions of the lung that are out of the irradiation field and that this effect is observable to a much greater extent in the apical region of the lung following irradiation of the base than in the base of the lung following irradiation of a similar volume of the apex. In this paper we describe an extension of these studies. We examined the effects of the irradiation of different regions of the lung on DNA damage detected in cells from regions both in and out of the radiation field. We demonstrate that DNA damage varies in different regions of the lung and is dependent both on the volume and region of the lung irradiated. Irradiation of partial volumes of the left or right lung base cause different levels of damage in out-of-field regions of the left and right quadrants of the apex and base of the rat lung, respectively.

5.2
Materials and Methods

Female Sprague-Dawley rats weighing 180–200 g were used in all the experiments. The animals were housed in animal facilities accredited by the Canadian Council on Animal Care and treated in accordance with approved protocols. Radiation-induced DNA damage was assessed using a well-characterized rat lung cell micronucleus assay [3]. Briefly, lungs of experimental rats were removed aseptically after perfusing them in situ with Hank's Balanced Salt Solution (HBSS; Sigma Chemical Co.). Following partial volume irradiation of the lung base, a strip of lung measuring 0.5 cm on either side of the expected field edge (superior/inferior) was removed as described previously [4], the remaining lung was divided into various regions and each lung piece was processed for analysis of micronucleus formation in the lung cells (primarily fibroblasts). The extent of DNA damage in the cells of the irradiated and shielded parts of the lungs was assessed by scoring the number of micronuclei (MN) per 1000 binucleate (BN) cells.

Detailed procedures for the whole lung or partial lung irradiation are described in our previous paper [4]. Briefly, a single dose of ^{60}Co gamma radiation (10 Gy) was delivered to the whole lung or to various regions of the lung. Lead blocks measuring 10 cm thick defined the irradiation field and shielded the adjacent tissue. Superior/inferior or lateral alignment of the field edge was determined for each rat by X-ray film localization using a portable diagnostic X-ray machine prior to each irradiation. For the whole lung irradiation, a field of 3 cm in length was defined from the position of the insertion of the second rib into the spine to below the dome of the diaphragm. From CT images (see below) this was determined to encompass the whole lung (98% +/− 3% of the lung volume) [4]. Shielding blocks were placed at 1.5 or 2.2 cm (superior/inferior) to shield or expose 30% upper/70% lung base or 70% upper/30% lung apex, respectively. In addition to blocks placed at 1.5 cm to shield the lung apex, extra lateral blocks were separately placed to shield regions of the lung base during partial irradiation of the left or right lung base. The effect of shielding block placement on the volume of lung irradiated was calculated using data from a series of axial computerized tomography (CT) images (1 mm thick) taken over the total lung region of seven rats (total of 16 complete scans), as described previously [4]. The relevant volumes are indicated in the figures and text.

5.3 Results

The results presented in Figure 5.1 show the effects of irradiation (10 Gy) of 30%, 70%, or 100% of the volume of the lung on DNA damage observed in different regions of the lung. Following irradiation of the whole lung there is significantly greater DNA damage observed in left lung than the right lung and in the base than in the apex. This effect is exacerbated when 70% of the lung volume is irradiated; the DNA damage in the irradiated lung base is similar to that observed when the whole lung is irradiated, but DNA damage in the irradiated lung apex is significantly reduced. When the lung base is irradiated, more DNA damage is observed in the left than the right base (see Table 5.1), similar to the results obtained following whole lung irradiation. When 30% of the lung volume is irradiated, the observed damage in the irradiated region of the base or apex is further reduced but is similar in both regions. Examination of DNA damage in shielded regions of the lungs following irradiation of 70% or 30% of

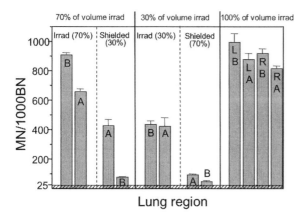

Fig. 5.1. DNA damage (micronuclei/1000 binucleate cells – MN/1000BN) observed in rat lung cells following a dose of 10 Gy given to different volumes of the lung base or lung apex. Cells from different regions of the lung were analysed (*B*, base; *A*, apex; *L*, left; *R*, right). The *bars* represent the mean (+/– SE) from groups of between four and seven rats. The hatched region at the bottom indicates the background level of micronuclei in non-irradiated rat lung; this does not vary for different regions of the lung, *irrad*, Irradiated

Table 5.1. DNA damage observed in different regions of the lungs of three different rats following a dose of 10 Gy to the lung base (70% of lung volume)

Lung region	Micronuclei/ 1000 binucleate cells			
	Left base	Left apex	Right base	Right apex
Rat 1	1150	448	974	174
Rat 2	1017	433	952	246
Rat 3	956	377	884	293
Mean	1041	419	937	238
(SE)	(57)	(22)	(27)	(35)

lung volume showed a substantial level of damage in the apex following irradiation of 70% volume in the lung base, but there was only a small effect for irradiation of 70% of the lung apex or 30% of the lung apex or base.

In the above studies we varied the volume irradiated by moving the lead shields in the superior/inferior (head to tail) direction and irradiated regions of both the left and right lung. Since there were different levels of DNA damage observed in the left and right lungs, and the out-of-field effect was most pronounced following irradiation of the lung base, we examined the effect of irradiating different volumes of the lung base using shields moved in the lateral (left-right) direction, while maintaining shielding of both apices. Results are shown in Figure 5.2 where the insets show the position of the irradiation field. The fields were not aligned to the spinal column (SC) because CT analysis demonstrated regions of the left and right lung lobes overlapping the midline. This overlap could extend up to 4 mm on either side, so the edge of the field was set at this position and expanded to include increasing volumes of the left or right base, as indicated in the inset figures. DNA damage was examined in the shielded left and right apices and in the irradiated left or right base. The analysis of the left and right base was only performed when the field included the complete base region. Lung regions given irradiation to part of their volume were not analysed. The results for the irradiated bases show a lower level of damage in the right base than the left base, as seen in the studies described above. The damage observed out-of-field, in the shielded apices, demonstrate an ipsilateral effect of the irradiation to the base and again show more damage if the left side is irradiated vs. the right side. When a small region encompassing an 8 mm strip across the midline of the lung base was irradiated, little or no damage above background (25 MN/1000 BN) was observed in either apex.

Further studies were then carried out to examine the effect of irradiating only the outer edges of the left or right lung base, as illustrated in Figure 5.3. Here the field was set to avoid irradiating any of the contralateral base and the analyses were confined to examining DNA damage in the shielded base or the two shielded apices. Very little damage was observed in any of three shielded regions, consistent with results shown in Figure 5.1 that out-of-field damage appears to be minimal if only a small volume of the lung is irradiated.

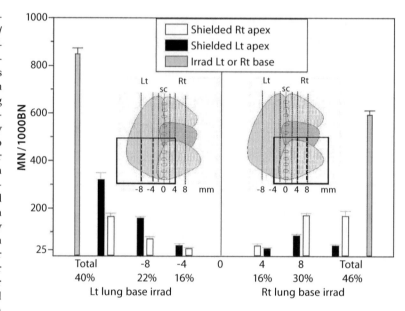

Fig. 5.2. DNA damage (micronuclei/1000 binucleate cells – MN/1000 BN) observed in cells from different regions of rat lung following irradiation (10 Gy) of different volumes of the left or right lung base. The *box* in the *insets* indicates the region of lung irradiated (*irrad*). Three different volumes were irradiated as indicated by the complete box (*Total*) or by the two *broken lines* at –4 mm and –8 mm for the left (*Lt*) lung and 4 mm and 8 mm for the right (*Rt*) lung. Estimated irradiated volumes, as a percent of the total lung volume, are indicated below each different position. The right boundary of the field for the left base irradiation and the left boundary of the field for the right base irradiation was fixed for the three different volumes. The upper boundary of the fields was fixed for all irradiations at the midpoint between the second rib insertion and the bottom of the lung (at 1.5 cm out of a total lung length of 3 cm). The bars represent the mean (+/– SE) from groups of four rats each

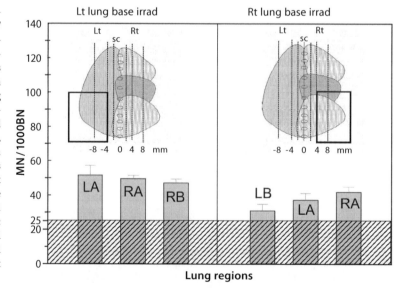

Fig. 5.3. DNA damage (micronuclei/1000 binucleate cells – MN/1000 BN) observed in cells from different regions of rat lung following irradiation (10 Gy) of different volumes of the left or right lung base. The *box* in the *insets* indicates the region of lung irradiated (*irrad*). Estimated irradiated volumes, as a percentage of total lung volume, were left (*Lt*) base, 24%, and right (*Rt*) base, 30%. Cells from three different regions of the lungs were analysed (*LA*, left apex; *RA*, right apex; *LB*, left base; *RB*, right base). The bars represent the mean (+/– SE) from groups of four rats. The *hatched region* at the *bottom* indicates the background level of micronuclei in non-irradiated rat lung; this does not vary for different regions of the lung

5.4 Discussion

The assay used in these studies measures DNA damage in individual cells and the irradiated or shielded regions of the lung are processed separately. Thus the differences in damage following irradiation of different volumes are not due to volume effects in the assay, as would be the case, for example, if a functional endpoint such as changes in breathing rate had been used. The results demonstrate a strong volume effect for this early measure of radiation-induced damage in the lung, both in terms of the region irradiated and the region analysed. Damage observed in-field is greater on the left side than the right side and greater in the base than in the apex. These results are in general agreement with our previous report and with the work of others, as discussed in Sect. 5.1 [1, 2, 4, 5, 7, 8].

Substantial out-of-field DNA damage is seen only when the lung base is irradiated and it is greater in the ipsilateral than in the contralateral apex. Detailed dosimetric analyses indicate that this regional damage on the ipsilateral side is much greater than what would be predicted by the out-of-field scatter dose. Irradiation of the left base causes greater damage than irradiation of the right base. The level of out-of-field DNA damage observed also depends strongly on the volume of the lung base that is irradiated; when this volume is 30% or less, very little out-of-field damage is observed. This very low level of damage may be due to scattered radiation; the dosimetric analyses demonstrate that levels of such scatter are quite low. Since the superior/inferior field edge was not altered during the irradiation of the different volumes of the lung base, scattered radiation is thus unlikely to explain the much greater level of damage observed when a larger volume of the lung base is irradiated.

We have suggested previously that the out-of-field DNA damage observed when the lung base is irradiated may reflect the action of an inflammatory response mounted in an effort to protect and repair the whole tissue. Since some of the DNA damage can be prevented by treating the animals with superoxide dismutase (SOD) or the nitric oxide synthase inhibitor L-nitro arginine methyl ester (L-NAME), these findings suggest the possibility that inflammatory cells are activated to produce reactive oxygen or nitroxyl species (ROS or RNS) that can cause DNA damage [4]. It has been reported that activated macrophages can be observed within 1 h of irradiation in lung tissue of C57Bl mice [9]. Early changes (within 6–24 h) in the level of the adhesion molecules ICAM-1 and E-selectin in lung endothelial cells have also been reported to occur following lung irradiation (2 Gy and larger), thereby increasing the arrest of inflammatory cells in the lung capillaries [10]. Mice knocked out for the ICAM-1 gene have been reported to be more resistant to the development of radiation-induced pneumonitis [10, 11]. The cells responsible for these various changes are believed to be primarily activated macrophages/monocytes.

Activation of these cells most probably occurs as a result of cytokine production in the lung following irradiation, which has been documented in many studies over the last 10 years. The early work of Rubin, Finkelstein and coworkers [12–15] demonstrated changes in mRNA levels for a number of inflammatory cytokines, in particular IL-1α, IL-1β, TNF-α, and TGF-β. They demonstrated changes within 1 day of irradiation (5 or 12.5 Gy) and found that the changes occurred in a cyclic pattern over the time period of the development of the symptoms described above. They postulated that these waves of cytokine expression preceded the development of the symptoms of radiation-induced pneumonitis and fibrosis. Others have confirmed that changes in mRNA levels of these cytokines can occur at very early times (within 1 h) and after quite low doses (~1 Gy), but the patterns of expression have not necessarily agreed between different studies, suggesting different patterns of response in different experimental systems [9, 16–20]. More recent studies have implicated changes in a much wider range of cytokines and chemokines following lung irradiation, although the extent to which such changes are a direct result of the radiation, as opposed to reactive changes associated with the changed expression of other cytokines and chemokines, remains to be established [21].

The generation of ROS and RNS will likely occur both in and out of the radiation field, thus we speculate that, while out-of-field damage will be caused primarily by such radicals, in-field DNA damage would be expected to be a combination of the direct effects of radiation on the cells plus the indirect effects of the ROS and RNS induced by the inflammatory response. The strong dependence of the out-of-field damage on volume and region irradiated implies that the extent of the inflammatory response depends on the volume and region of the lung that is irradiated. A greater inflammatory response is generated if the base is irradiated, particularly if it is the left base. This concept can explain why differences in the amount of in-field damage are observed depending on the volume and region irradiated. These differences might reflect the different contributions of the indirect effect of the induced inflammatory response.

Regardless of the mechanism of the volume effects that we have demonstrated, such effects have substantial implications for attempts to model normal tissue complication probabilities (NTCP) based on dose-volume histograms (DVH). Our results and those of others argue strongly that simple application of DVH analysis without consideration of the region of lung irradiated is likely to be problematic for predicting lung complications following radiotherapy. Recent clinical data published by Yorke et al. [22] demonstrate trends in human lungs that are consistent with our laboratory results in rodents. Additional clinical data and more detailed analyses of the complications arising when similar volumes of different regions of the human lung are irradiated should help to clarify this important issue.

Acknowledgements:

This work is supported by a grant from the Ontario Cancer Research Network.

References

1. Liao ZX, Travis EL, Tucker SL (1995) Damage and morbidity from pneumonitis after irradiation of partial volumes of mouse lung. Int J Radiat Oncol Biol Phys 32:1359–1370
2. Travis EL, Liao ZX, Tucker SL (1997) Spatial heterogeneity of the volume effect for radiation pneumonitis in mouse lung. Int J Radiat Oncol Biol Phys 38:1045–1054
3. Khan MA, Hill RP, Van Dyk J (1998) Partial volume rat lung irradiation: an evaluation of early DNA damage. Int J Radiat Oncol Biol Phys 40:467–476
4. Khan MA, Van Dyk J, Yeung IW et al (2003) Partial volume rat lung irradiation; assessment of early DNA damage in different lung regions and effect of radical scavengers. Radiother Oncol 66:95–102
5. Wiegman EM, Meertens H, Konings AW et al (2003) Locoregional differences in pulmonary function and density after partial rat lung irradiation. Radiother Oncol 69:11–19
6. Tucker SL, Liao ZX, Travis EL (1997) Estimation of the spatial distribution of target cells for radiation pneumonitis in mouse lung. Int J Radiat Oncol Biol Phys 38:1055–1066
7. Herrmann T, Baumann M, Voigtmann L et al (1997) Effect of irradiated volume on lung damage in pigs. Radiother Oncol 44:35–40
8. Baumann M, Appold S, Geyer P et al (2000) Lack of effect of small high-dose volumes on the dose-response relationship for the development of fibrosis in distant parts of the ipsilateral lung in mini-pigs. Int J Radiat Biol 76:477–485
9. Rube CE, Uthe D, Schmid KW et al (2000) Dose-dependent induction of transforming growth factor beta (TGF-beta) in the lung tissue of fibrosis-prone mice after thoracic irradiation. Int J Radiat Oncol Biol Phys 47:1033–1042
10. Hallahan DE, Virudachalam S (1997) Ionizing radiation mediates expression of cell adhesion molecules in distinct histological patterns within the lung. Cancer Res 57:2096–2099
11. Hallahan DE, Geng L, Shyr Y (2002) Effects of intercellular adhesion molecule 1 (ICAM-1) null mutation on radiation-induced pulmonary fibrosis and respiratory insufficiency in mice. J Natl Cancer Inst 94:733–741
12. Johnston CJ, Piedboeuf B, Baggs R et al (1995) Differences in correlation of mRNA gene expression in mice sensitive and resistant to radiation-induced pulmonary fibrosis. Radiat Res 142:197–203
13. Johnston CJ, Piedboeuf B, Rubin P et al (1996) Early and persistent alterations in the expression of interleukin-1 alpha, interleukin-1 beta and tumor necrosis factor alpha mRNA levels in fibrosis-resistant and sensitive mice after thoracic irradiation. Radiat Res 145:762–767
14. Johnston CJ, Wright TW, Rubin P et al (1998) Alterations in the expression of chemokine mRNA levels in fibrosis-resistant and -sensitive mice after thoracic irradiation. Exp Lung Res 24:321–337
15. Rubin P, Johnston CJ, Williams JP et al (1995) A perpetual cascade of cytokines postirradiation leads to pulmonary fibrosis. Int J Radiat Oncol Biol Phys 33:99–109
16. Rube CE, Wilfert F, Uthe D et al (2002) Modulation of radiation-induced tumour necrosis factor alpha (TNF-alpha) expression in the lung tissue by pentoxifylline. Radiother Oncol 64:177–187
17. Hong JH, Chiang CS, Tsao CY et al (1999) Rapid induction of cytokine gene expression in the lung after single and fractionated doses of radiation. Int J Radiat Biol 75:1421–1427
18. Hong JH, Chiang CS, Tsao CY et al (2001) Can short-term administration of dexamethasone abrogate radiation-induced acute cytokine gene response in lung and modify subsequent molecular responses? Int J Radiat Oncol Biol Phys 51:296–303
19. Yi ES, Bedoya A, Lee H et al (1996) Radiation-induced lung injury in vivo: expression of transforming growth factor-beta precedes fibrosis. Inflammation 20:339–352
20. Vujaskovic Z, Batinic-Haberle I, Rabbani ZN, et al (2002) A small molecular weight catalytic metalloporphyrin antioxidant with superoxide dismutase (SOD) mimetic properties protects lungs from radiation-induced injury. Free Radic Biol Med 33:857–863
21. Johnston CJ, Williams JP, Okunieff P et al (2002) Radiation-induced pulmonary fibrosis: examination of chemokine and chemokine receptor families. Radiat Res 157:256–265
22. Yorke ED, Jackson A, Rosenzweig KE et al (2002) Dose-volume factors contributing to the incidence of radiation pneumonitis in non-small-cell lung cancer patients treated with three-dimensional conformal radiation therapy. Int J Radiat Oncol Biol Phys 54:329–339

The Role of Imaging in the Study of Radiation-Induced Normal Tissue Injury

ZAFER KOCAK, LALITHA SHANKAR, DANIEL C. SULLIVAN, and LAWRENCE B. MARKS

CONTENTS

6.1 Introduction 38
6.2 Lung Injury 38
6.3 Heart Injury 41
6.4 Brain Injury 42
6.5 Salivary Glands 42
6.6 Clinical Relevance 43
6.7 Conclusions 43
References 44

Summary

The recognition and assessment of normal tissue injury is an important aspect of radiation oncology practice and a critical endpoint in clinical studies. One of the major challenges in the study of radiation (RT)-induced normal tissue injury is determining the appropriate endpoint. Patients' symptoms have obvious clinical relevance; however, the scoring of symptoms is relatively subjective. Conversely, radiologic endpoints are potentially quantifiable and are available for objective study. Furthermore, radiologic evidence of subclinical normal tissue injury is far more common than are clinical symptoms, providing a larger number of patients with identifiable injury for study. We review herein radiologically-detected normal tissue injury as it relates to the lung, heart, brain, and salivary glands. The concepts described are likely to be similar for other organs. We conclude that:

(1) radiologically-defined normal tissue injury in human patients may be related to long-term, clinically meaningful injury, but further study is needed to better quantify this association;

(2) radiologically-defined normal tissue injury in human patients is manifest soon after (or even during) RT and hence is a potential tool to rapidly study potential mitigators of this injury in humans; and

(3) additional work is needed to develop standards to quantitatively score radiologic injury. Thus, advances in anatomic and functional imaging afford unique opportunities to facilitate the study of radiation-associated normal tissue injury.

Z. KOCAK, MD
Department of Radiation Oncology, Duke University Medical Center, Box 3085, Durham, NC 27710, USA
and
Department of Radiation Oncology, Trakya University Hospital, Edirne, 22030, Turkey

L. SHANKAR, MD,PhD
D. C. SULLIVAN, MD,PhD
Biomedical Imaging Program, National Cancer Institute, EPN, Room 6070, 6130 Executive Blvd, Rockville, MD 20892–7412, USA

L. B. MARKS, MD
Professor, Department of Radiation Oncology, Duke University Medical Center, Box 3085, Durham, NC 27710, USA

6.1 Introduction

One of the major challenges in the study of radiation (RT)-induced normal tissue injury is determining the appropriate endpoint. Patients' symptoms have obvious clinical relevance. However, the scoring of symptoms is relatively subjective. Conversely, radiologic endpoints are quantifiable and are readily available for objective study. Furthermore, radiologic evidence of subclinical normal tissue injury is far more common than are clinical symptoms, providing a larger number of patients with identifiable injury for study. The choice of endpoint is critical as it has a large impact on the reported incidence of organ injury. Using the lung as an example, Table 7.1 illustrates several of the different available endpoints, divided based on subjective vs. objective, and regional vs. global. In this chapter, we will focus on the regional/objective quadrant of Table 7.1 as it relates to the lung, heart, brain, and salivary glands. The concepts described are likely to be similar for other organs.

Table 6.1. Different types of endpoints that can be used to study RT-induced lung injury, organized on the basis of clinical vs. subclinical and regional vs. global assessments

	Endpoints for RT-induced lung injury	
	Regional	Global
Clinical		Shortness of breath, cough
Subclinical	Radiologic (computed tomography, perfusion/ventilation scans)	Pulmonary function tests, exercise testing

6.2 Lung Injury

The frequency of detecting radiologic abnormalities depends on the sensitivity of the radiographic assessment used. The data from many studies are summarized in Table 6.2 [1–5]. Increases in tissue density, associated with acute inflammation or late fibrosis, are typically seen on either chest radiograph or computed tomography (CT) scan within several months of RT [6]. CT is more sensitive than chest radiography because it provides better three-dimensional (3D) visualization of the lung. By 24 months, most patients receiving moderate to high doses of RT have radiologic evidence of lung fibrosis, often manifested by lung contraction, plural thickening, tenting of the diaphragm, and deviation of trachea or mediastinum toward the irradiated region. The incidence of radiographic change is related to dose of RT [7] and, perhaps, the use/intensity of chemotherapy [8, 9].

Several investigators have related lung doses to CT-defined lung injury [2, 6, 10]. Mah et al. prospectively studied changes in CT density 6 months or earlier following lung irradiation in a series of 54 patients [2]. They demonstrated a dose–response relationship between the frequency of finding CT evidence of lung injury and the estimated single dose from the nominal standard dose model. That particular study considered the frequency of a radiologic abnormality, and not the severity of the abnormality.

Investigators at Duke and the Netherlands Cancer Institute (NKI) have formally studied this issue using 3D image fusion techniques to relate changes

Table 6.2. The frequency of radiographic changes and symptoms following thoracic irradiation

Reference	Author Year	No. of cases	Disease	Follow-up	Assay	Frequency of imaging abnormality (%)	Frequency of symptomatic cases (%)
[2]	Mah (1987)	54	Lung, breast, Hodgkin's	6 months	Computed Tomography	36/54 (67%)	10/54 (19%)
[5]	Rotstein (1990)	33	Breast	9 months	Computed Tomography	24/33 (73%)	13/33 (39%)
[4]	Polansky (1980)	37	Breast	0.7–10 years	Chest X-ray	16/37 (43%)	0/37 (0%)
[1]	Allevena (1992)	75	Hodgkin's	3–10 years	Chest X-ray Ventilation Perfusion	12/75 (16%) 0/45 (0%) 29/45 (64%)	0/45 (0%)
[3]	Marks (2000)	184	Lung, breast, lymphoma	24 months	Perfusion Computed Tomography	186/230 (81%) 162/259 (63%)	34/175 (19%)

between the pre- and post-RT images to the 3D dose distribution. Using this approach, one can study the dose-dependent nature of this regional injury since different regions of the lung receive different doses of RT (Fig. 6.1). At Duke, changes in local CT density were studied in 13 patients with lung cancer [6]. Marked increases in CT density were seen in lung regions receiving >60 Gy, with variable/modest changes seen at lower doses. The pre- and post-RT CT images for a typical patient irradiated for lung cancer are shown in Figure 6.2. The course of the RT beam is shown. In 25 patients who were irradiated for malignant lymphoma at the NKI, Boersma and colleagues observed a dose-dependent increase in CT density 3–4 months post-RT, followed by only a slight change at 18 months [10].

Nuclear medicine imaging provides a sensitive means to assess regional lung function. Single photon emission computed tomography (SPECT) perfusion and ventilation scans provide a 3D map of perfusion and ventilation. As is described above for CT images, the pre- and post-RT SPECT images can be compared, in the context of the 3D dose distribution, to study the dose-dependent nature of this regional injury. The pre- and post-RT SPECT perfusion images from a patient irradiated for lung cancer are shown in Figure 6.3. The isodose distribution is included.

The study cited above from the Netherlands Cancer Institute by Boersma et al. also considered changes in regional SPECT perfusion and ventilation 3 and 18 months post-RT in the same 25 patients with malignant lymphoma [10]. They reported dose-dependent reductions in both ventilation and perfusion at 3–4 months, followed by a 50%–60% partial recovery at 18 months. In a similar study of 110 patients irradiated for breast cancer and lymphoma, Theuws et al. also reported dose-dependent reductions in ventilation and regional perfusion at 3 months, followed by 10%–50% partial recovery

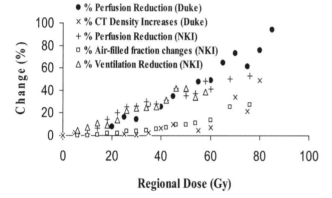

Fig. 6.1. Dose-dependent reductions in regional SPECT perfusion and ventilation, and increases in CT density in humans. (Adapted from [50] with permission) (data from Netherlands Cancer Institute, NKI, [13] and Duke [6,12])

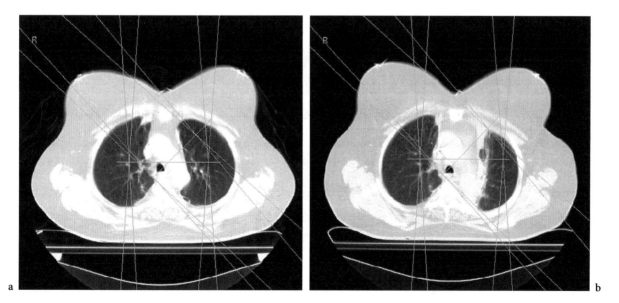

Fig. 6.2a,b. The pre- and 12-month post-RT CT images from a patient irradiated for lung cancer are shown in (a) and (b), respectively. The beam paths are shown (anterior, posterior, oblique). There is increased CT density in the irradiated medial left lung following RT

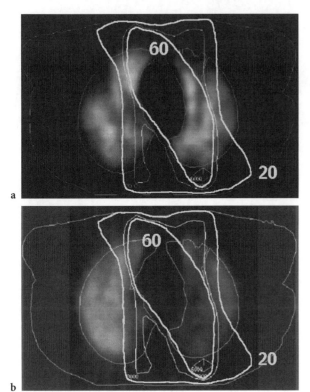
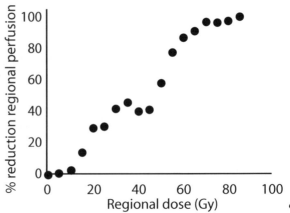

Fig. 6.3a–c. The pre- and 6-month post-RT transverse SPECT perfusion images from a patient irradiated for lung cancer are shown (above and below, respectively). The RT dose distribution is also shown. The post-RT perfusion defect is seen most prominently within regions of the lung receiving > 60 Gy. The dose–response curve for RT-induced reductions in regional perfusion, from this patient's SPECT scans, is shown

at 18 months, without further change at 48 months [11]. In the Netherlands data, perfusion appears to be more sensitive than ventilation, and both are more sensitive than CT. This appears to be best appreciated in the modest dose range (~15–40 Gy) when there often is no change seen in tissue density, yet reductions in both ventilation and perfusion are evident (Fig. 6.1). From Duke, Woel et al. reported progressive, dose-dependent reductions in regional perfusion 3–24 months post-RT, with most (80%) of the ultimate damage manifest within 12 months post-RT [12]. The progression of perfusion injury over time occurred mostly within regions of the lung exposed to > 50 Gy. Recovery of regional perfusion over time was not observed. This might be due to the higher RT doses used in these lung cancer patients vs. the lower doses reported in the breast and lymphoma patients reported from the NKI.

The Netherlands group compared the regional dose–effect relation in 25 patients with lung cancer (i.e. "unhealthy lungs") to that seen in 81 patients with breast cancer and lymphoma (i.e. "healthy lungs") [13]. They report that well-perfused lung regions of lung within lung-cancer patients showed the same dose-effect relationship as the healthy-lung in the breast/lymphoma group. These results support the concept that regional injury in a parallel-structured organ such as the lung is relatively independent of the physiologic state of other regions. In the poorly perfused regions of the lung in the lung-cancer patients, reperfusion (likely due to tumor shrinkage) was noted on the post-RT scan in 18 of 25 patients.

The changes in magnetic resonance imaging (MRI) signal following radiation are not well described. However, MRI may be more sensitive than chest X-ray and possibly CT scans [14]. Yankelevitz et al. evaluated the treatment response of ten consecutive patients with lung cancer by using MRI before and after RT. They found that the irradiated lung parenchyma had increased signal on both the T1- and T2-weighted images as early as 17 days after the start of RT. The signal intensity continued to increase over the first 6 months post-RT, but subsequently decreased.

What is the clinical relevance of radiologically-detected regional lung injury? In an organ with a parallel architecture like the lung, it is logical to hypothesize that the sum of regional injuries (e.g. the integrated response) will be equal to, or at least related to, changes in whole organ function. Investigators at Duke and the NKI have demonstrated that the integrated response in the lung is statistically related to declines in pulmonary function tests ($P \approx 0.002-0.24$) [15, 16], though the correlation coefficients are suboptimal ($r \approx 0.20-0.70$). The integrated response is highly correlated with dosimetric parameters (e.g., mean lung dose, percent of lung receiving ≥ 20 Gy), and they are all related to the risk of developing pulmonary symptoms [17–21].

6.3
Heart Injury

RT to the thorax may induce both early and late cardiac effects if portions of the heart are included in the radiation field. Breast cancer and Hodgkin's disease patients are particularly at risk for developing late myocardial damage, due to their longevity and the frequent use of anthracycline-containing chemotherapy. In general, one has to wait many years to see these effects manifest clinically. Radiologic methods allow for the early detection of treatment-associated dysfunction. The full spectrum of therapy-associated heart injury is discussed elsewhere in this book [22].

Seddon et al. performed SPECT myocardial perfusion imaging in 24 patients with left-breast tumors, and 12 control patients with right-breast tumors, who had undergone RT at least 5 years previously [23]. Myocardial perfusion defects were found in 17/24 (70.8%) of left-breast patients vs. 2/12 (16.7%) of right-breast patients. Almost all myocardial defects in left-breast patients were located in the cardiac apex (the portion of heart that is incidentally included within the RT fields). Gyenes et al. conducted a prospective study and performed Tc-99m Sestamibi scintigraphy prior to and approximately 1 year after left breast/chest wall RT in 12 patients [24]. Six of 12 patients (50%) with some left ventricle within the radiation field exhibited a new perfusion defect. Again, the location of the defects corresponded with the irradiated volume of the left ventricle. Interestingly, neither electrocardiographic changes nor left ventricular segmental wall motion abnormalities were detected by echocardiography [25].

In a prospective study from Duke, new RT-associated perfusion defects were detected in 16/55 (29%) patients 6–12 months post-RT. The incidence is related to the volume of left ventricle irradiated with new defects occurring in approximately 10%–20% and 50%–60% of patients with <5% and >5% of their left ventricle included within the RT fields, respectively [26]. Furthermore, such perfusion defects are associated with episodes of chest pain [27], and wall motion abnormalities [28]. This literature is summarized in the Table 6.3 [23–25, 29–31]. These data suggest that radiologically-detected abnormalities in regional function are clinically significant. In the study by Marks [28], there were minimal, if any reductions in ejection fraction associated with these perfusion defects. This may be explained by the small irradiated volumes in most patients. Perfusion defects need to involve relatively large fractions of the heart to affect ejection fraction [32]. Furthermore, the increased risk for ischemic cardiac disease may be observed only in patients with known cardiovascular risk factors [33, 34]. MRI has been suggested as a sensitive means to assess myocardial injury in patients with coronary artery disease [35]. This approach has not been applied to the study of RT-induced cardiac disease.

Table 6.3. Summary of studies using myocardial perfusion scintigraphy to detect RT-induced cardiac injury in patients irradiated for left breast cancer

Reference	Author (Year)	Years of RT	No. of patients	Follw-up (years)	Rate of perfusion defects
[24]	Gyenes (1994)	1971–1976	37	18.4	25% (5/20)
[30]	Hojris (2000)	1982–1990	16	7.9	44% (4/9)[a]
[29]	Cowen (1998)	1987–1993	17	8.4	0% (0/17)
[23]	Seddon (2002)	1987–1995	36	6.7	71% (17/24)[b]
[25]	Gyenes (1996)	1993–1994	12	1.1	50% (6/12)
[31]	Marks (2005)	1998–2001	114	2	42% (11/26)

[a] Similar rate of perfusion defects (4/7) seen in unirradiated patients.
[b] Lower rate of perfusion defects (2/12) seen in patients irradiated for right-sided lesions.

6.4
Brain Injury

The infiltrative nature of gliomas necessitates adjuvant therapy following surgical tumor debulking. Currently, radiation therapy is one of the few effective therapeutic options available. However, the prognosis for a malignant glioma is poor, with 90% of recurring tumors occurring in the primary tumor bed. A significant factor contributing to this poor prognosis has been the dose restrictions required in routine external radiation due to the significant complications of edema, radiation necrosis and brain atrophy [36]. Methods, which utilize high dose rate radiation in a limited treatment volume, include stereotactic radiosurgery and brachytherapy.

There is significant overlap in the radiologic findings seen in recurrent neoplasm and therapy-induced abnormalities primarily due the alterations in the blood–brain barrier that is present in both situations. The diagnostic modalities available, in varying levels of maturation in neuroimaging, include CT, conventional MRI, perfusion (dynamic contrast enhancement, DCE) MRI, magnetic resonance spectroscopy, diffusion weighted MRI, positron emission tomography (PET), and SPECT.

Mishima et al. compared CT and MRI in a primate model of radiation-induced brain injury [36]. They applied iridium-192 interstitial irradiation to the brains of 14 normal monkeys and followed them periodically over 6 months post-irradiation with CT and MRI. MRI performed better than CT in their study, revealing a focus of necrosis, with peripheral ring enhancement and edema 1 week after therapy. They reported transient improvement radiographically at 4 weeks, with worsening and persistence for as long as 6 months.

To image functional changes, there has been extensive work performed using both SPECT and PET nuclear medicine imaging techniques in evaluating the effects of radiation therapy on brain tumors.

Fluorodeoxyglucose (FDG) uptake in a tumor generally decreases in tumors responding to therapy. FDG-PET scans are usually performed several weeks after the completion of therapy to allow the abatement of inflammatory components induced by radiation [37]. Moreover, studies have documented an increase in FDG uptake in brain tumors in the hours after radiation therapy. It is postulated that this increase in glucose metabolism may represent an energy-dependent "acute rescue system" in tumor cells or be due to the influx of inflammatory cells. This upregulation in glucose utilization is also thought to be secondary to the energy-dependent radiation repair processes and enhanced apoptosis [38, 39].

SPECT, using a variety of radiopharmaceuticals such as 3-[123I] iodo-alpha-methyl- L-tyrosine (IMT), thallium-201, and 99mTc-MIBI, has shown varying degrees of success in differentiating between recurrent tumor and radiation necrosis [40, 41]. Hein et al. have shown that it may be possible to use diffusion weighted magnetic resonance, by employing the differences in the apparent diffusion co-efficient of different morphologic features such as edema, necrosis, and tumor tissue, to differentiate between recurrent tumor and radiation necrosis [42].

Walecki et al. have observed changes in magnetic resonance spectroscopy without concomitant changes in the magnetic resonance images, presumably due to the improved sensitivity of the former methodology to detect the early metabolic effects of therapy [43]. Choline related ratios, as opposed to creatine, may prove to be more specific for cell proliferation, indicative of recurrent tumor. Thus, at the present time, there is no single anatomic or functional imaging test that can reliably sort out the effects of radiation on tumor vs. the surrounding brain tissue.

6.5
Salivary Glands

Salivary glands may be injured by radiation from external radiation therapy for head and neck tumors, or from I-131 administrated for thyroid cancer therapy. The management of differentiated thyroid cancer often involves administration of a therapeutic (ablative) dose of radioactive iodine (I-131) after sub-total thyroidectomy. The salivary parenchyma consequently undergoes dose-related damage from the I-131 therapy. Alexander et al. studied 203 patients within 3 months of I-131 therapy (100–200 mCi) and found that 67 patients (33%) had symptoms of sialadenitis, often bilateral [44]. Patients were prophylactically administered sialogogic agents, whose effects have not been studied in a prospective fashion.

The objective evaluation of salivary gland function can be accomplished by measuring saliva production and by dynamic scintigraphic examination using technetium-99m pertechnetate [45]. The latter yields information related to the uptake, concentration, and the excretory phase of salivation. Thus, information regarding the effects of irradiation on the different phases of gland activity can be obtained. Scintigraphy results have a reasonable correlation with salivary output measurements [46]. Scintigraphy, especially when combined with SPECT, provides spatial information about the anatomical gland volumes and their response to the variation of doses within the gland, information that cannot be provided by other methods [47].

There is a documented association between radiation exposure dose and the risk of developing a salivary gland tumor, both after external beam radiation therapy to the head and neck region, as well as after I-131 therapy for thyroid cancer [48]. A small but statistically significant rise in salivary gland tumors has been noted. Developments of pleomorphic adenoma, Hodgkin's lymphoma, and mucoepidermoid carcinoma have been reported [44, 45, 48]. These secondary cancers are best imaged with CT or MRI.

MRI has also been used to quantify RT-induced salivary gland injury. Zhang et al. noted a reduction in MRI-defined apparent diffusion coefficient in patients with RT-induced dysfunction as assessed by scintigraphy [49].

6.6 Clinical Relevance

The importance of subclinical radiologic regional injury in scoring treatment-related side effects is certainly questionable. The A of the SOMA/LENT system reflects such analytic data, and hence acknowledges it's potential role in "scoring" late effects. The importance of the analytic component needs to be taken in the context of the overall clinical situation and competing risks. For example, in patients irradiated for unresectable lung cancer, asymptomatic lung injury should be of little concern since the competing risk of disease-related morbidity and death is high. Conversely, in patients irradiated post-operatively for lung cancer or for breast cancer, where the disease-specific survival is better, subclinical injury of the lung or heart may be a marker for subsequent clinical sequelae, and hence may be relatively more important.

Historically, prospective studies involving late effects, by definition, need to have relatively long follow-up. This is expensive and often impractical. Tremendous advances in imaging afford a unique opportunity to detect and study treatment-induced organ injury long before the toxicity is manifest clinically. Agents that mitigate such injury can be tested directly in human patients, and the radiologic endpoints provide objective data within a relatively short interval. Thus, radiologically-defined injury is a potentially useful research tool in clinical oncology. Prospective studies to develop and exploit these tools should be conducted.

The approach described above assumes that such radiologic injury is clinically-relevant. We believe that it is. However, additional work is clearly needed to better understand the relationship between subclinical radiologic injury and clinically-relevant events. This will require lengthy clinical trials in human patients. Large numbers of patients likely need to be enrolled onto such studies in order to have an ample number of patients evaluable at longer time points. This work is difficult but possible. We believe that important questions in late-effects research can be explored through the careful prospective and systematic study of human patients.

Radiographic studies provide objective quantitative data regarding RT-induced normal tissue injury. However, there are several challenges that remain. There are presently no well-accepted standards to how one evaluates a radiograph. If a degree of radiographic injury is different within different regions of an organ, does one report the average radiographic abnormality, the maximum, etc.? Do we report the absolute increase in lung density seen by CT, or do we report it as percent change from baseline?

In many ways, the radiographic endpoints suffer from the same potential ambiguities as do the clinical endpoints (e.g., do we score the maximum severity of the patient's diarrhea, or the duration of diarrhea?). To make this work fruitful, standards on how to report such radiologic abnormalities need to be developed.

6.7 Conclusions

- Radiologically-defined normal tissue injury in human patients may be related to long-term

clinically meaningful injury, but further study is needed to better quantify this association.
- Radiologically-defined normal tissue injury in human patients is manifest soon after (or even during) RT and hence may be a powerful tool for early detection of normal tissue injury, and for study of potential mitigators of this injury in humans.
- Additional work is needed to develop methods and standards to quantitatively score radiologic injury.

References

1. Allavena C, Conroy T, Aletti P et al (1992) Late cardiopulmonary toxicity after treatment for Hodgkin's disease. Br J Cancer 65:908–912
2. Mah K, Van Dyk J, Keane T et al (1987) Acute radiation-induced pulmonary damage: a clinical study on the response to fractionated radiation therapy. Int J Radiat Oncol Biol Phys 13:179–188
3. Marks LB, Fan M, Clough R et al (2000) Radiation-induced pulmonary injury: symptomatic versus subclinical endpoints. Int J Radiat Biol 76:469–475
4. Polansky SM, Ravin CE, Prosnitz LR (1980) Pulmonary changes after primary irradiation for early breast carcinoma. AJR Am J Roentgenol 134:101–105
5. Rotstein S, Lax I, Svane G (1990) Influence of radiation therapy on the lung-tissue in breast cancer patients: CT-assessed density changes and associated symptoms. Int J Radiat Oncol Biol Phys 18:173–180
6. Levinson B, Marks LB, Munley MT et al (1998) Regional dose response to pulmonary irradiation using a manual method. Radiother Oncol 48:53–60
7. Rosen II, Fischer TA, Antolak JA et al (2001) Correlation between lung fibrosis and radiation therapy dose after concurrent radiation therapy and chemotherapy for limited small cell lung cancer. Radiology 221:614–622
8. Theuws JC, Kwa SL, Wagenaar AC et al (1998) Dose-effect relations for early local pulmonary injury after irradiation for malignant lymphoma and breast cancer. Radiother Oncol 48:33–43
9. Trask CW, Joannides T, Harper PG et al (1985) Radiation-induced lung fibrosis after treatment of small cell carcinoma of the lung with very high-dose cyclophosphamide. Cancer 55:57–60
10. Boersma LJ, Damen EM, de Boer RW et al (1996) Recovery of overall and local lung function loss 18 months after irradiation for malignant lymphoma. J Clin Oncol 14:1431–141
11. Theuws JC, Seppenwoolde Y, Kwa SL et al (2000) Changes in local pulmonary injury up to 48 months after irradiation for lymphoma and breast cancer. Int J Radiat Oncol Biol Phys 47:1201–1208
12. Woel RT, Munley MT, Hollis D et al (2002) The time course of radiation therapy-induced reductions in regional perfusion: a prospective study with > 5 years of follow-up. Int J Radiat Oncol Biol Phys 52:58–67
13. Seppenwoolde Y, Muller SH, Theuws JC et al. (2000) Radiation dose-effect relations and local recovery in perfusion for patients with non-small-cell lung cancer. Int J Radiat Oncol Biol Phys 47:681–690
14. Yankelevitz DF, Henschke CI, Batata M et al. (1994) Lung cancer: evaluation with MR imaging during and after irradiation. J Thorac Imaging 9:41–46
15. Boersma LJ, Damen EM, de Boer RW et al (1996) Estimation of overall pulmonary function after irradiation using dose-effect relations for local functional injury. Radiother Oncol 36:15–23
16. Fan M, Marks LB, Lind P et al (2001) Relating radiation-induced regional lung injury to changes in pulmonary function tests. Int J Radiat Oncol Biol Phys 51:311–317
17. Graham MV, Purdy JA, Emami B et al (1999) Clinical dose-volume histogram analysis for pneumonitis after 3D treatment for non-small cell lung cancer (NSCLC). Int J Radiat Oncol Biol Phys 45:323–329
18. Kwa SL, Lebesque JV, Theuws JC et al (1998) Radiation pneumonitis as a function of mean lung dose: an analysis of pooled data of 540 patients. Int J Radiat Oncol Biol Phys 42:1–9
19. Lind PA, Marks LB, Hollis D et al (2002) Receiver operating characteristic curves to assess predictors of radiation-induced symptomatic lung injury. Int J Radiat Oncol Biol Phys 54:340–347
20. Martel MK, Ten Haken RK, Hazuka MB et al (1994) Dose-volume histogram and 3-D treatment planning evaluation of patients with pneumonitis. Int J Radiat Oncol Biol Phys 28:575–581
21. Oetzel D, Schraube P, Hensley F et al (1995) Estimation of pneumonitis risk in three-dimensional treatment planning using dose-volume histogram analysis. Int J Radiat Oncol Biol Phys 33:455–460
22. Adams MJ, Prosnitz RG, Constine LS, Marks LB, Lipshultz SE (2006) Screening for cardiovascular disease in survivors of thoracic radiation. Sem Rad Onc, in press
23. Seddon B, Cook A, Gothard L et al (2002) Detection of defects in myocardial perfusion imaging in patients with early breast cancer treated with radiotherapy. Radiother Oncol 64:53–63
24. Gyenes G, Fornander T, Carlens P (1994) Morbidity of ischemic heart disease in early breast cancer 15–20 years after adjuvant radiotherapy. Int J Radiat Oncol Biol Phys 28:1235–1241
25. Gyenes G, Fornander T, Carlens P et al (1996) Myocardial damage in breast cancer patients treated with adjuvant radiotherapy: a prospective study. Int J Radiat Oncol Biol Phys 36:899–905
26. Marks LB, Yu XL, Zhou SM et al (2003) The incidence and functional consequences of RT-associated cardiac perfusion defects. Int J Radiat Oncol Biol Phys. 2005 Sep 1;63(1):214–223
27. Yu X, Prosnitz RR, Zhou S et al (2003) Symptomatic cardiac events following radiation therapy for left-sided breast cancer: possible association with radiation therapy-induced changes in regional perfusion. Clin Breast Cancer 4:193–197
28. Marks LB, Prosnitz RB, Hardenbergh PM et al (2002) Functional consequences of radiation (RT)-induced per-

fusion changes in patients with left-sided breast cancer. Int J Radiat Oncol Biol Phys 54:S3-4
29. Cowen D, Gonzague-Casabianca L, Brenot-Rossi I et al (1998) Thallium-201 perfusion scintigraphy in the evaluation of late myocardial damage in left-side breast cancer treated with adjuvant radiotherapy. Int J Radiat Oncol Biol Phys 41:809-815
30. Hojris I, Sand NP, Andersen J et al (2000) Myocardial perfusion imaging in breast cancer patients treated with or without post-mastectomy radiotherapy. Radiother Oncol 55:163-172
31. Marks LB, Yu X, Prosnitz RG et al (2005) The incidence and functional consequences of RT-associated cardiac perfusion defects. Int J Radiat Oncol Biol Phys 63:214-223
32. Borges-Neto S, Coleman RE, Potts JM et al (1991) Combined exercise radionuclide angiocardiography and single photon emission computed tomography perfusion studies for assessment of coronary artery disease. Semin Nucl Med 21:223-229
33. Glanzmann C, Kaufmann P, Jenni R et al (1998) Cardiac risk after mediastinal irradiation for Hodgkin's disease. Radiother Oncol 46:51-62
34. Gustavsson A, Bendahl PO, Cwikiel M et al (1999) No serious late cardiac effects after adjuvant radiotherapy following mastectomy in premenopausal women with early breast cancer. Int J Radiat Oncol Biol Phys 43:745-754
35. Li D, Desphande V (2001) Magnetic resonance imaging of coronary arteries. Top Magn Reson Imaging 12:337-347
36. Mishima N, Tamiya T, Matsumoto K et al (2003) Radiation damage to the normal monkey brain: experimental study induced by interstitial irradiation. Acta Med Okayama 57:123-131
37. Ogawa T, Uemura K, Shishido F et al (1988) Changes of cerebral blood flow, and oxygen and glucose metabolism following radiochemotherapy of gliomas: a PET study. J Comput Assist Tomogr. 12:290-297
38. Maruyama I, Sadato N, Waki A et al (1999) Hyperacute changes in glucose metabolism of brain tumors after stereotactic radiosurgery: a PET study. J Nucl Med 40:1085-1090

39. Spence A, Muzi M, Graham MM et al (2002) 2 (18F) Fluoro-2-deoxyglucose and glucose uptake in malignant gliomas before and after radiotherapy: correlation with outcome. Clin Cancer Res 8:971-979
40. Henze M, Mohammed A, Schlemmer H et al (2002) Detection of tumor progression in the follow-up of irradiated low-grade astrocytomas: comparison of 3-[123I]iodo-alpha-methyl- L-tyrosine and 99mTc-MIBI SPET. Eur J Nucl Med Mol Imaging 29:1455-1461
41. Vos MJ, Hoekstra OS, Barkhof F et al (2003) Thallium-201 single-photon emission computed tomography as an early predictor of outcome in recurrent glioma. J Clin Oncol 21:3559-3565
42. Hein P, Eskey C, Dunn JE et al (2004) Diffusion-weighted imaging in the follow-up of treated high-grade gliomas: tumor recurrence versus radiation injury. AJNR Am J Neuroradiol 25:201-209
43. Walecki J, Sokol M, Pieniazek P et al (1999) Role of short TE 1H-MR spectroscopy in the monitoring of post-operation irradiated patients. Eur J Rad 30:154-161
44. Alexander C, Bader JB, Schaefer A et al (1998) Intermediate and long-term side effects of high dose radioiodine therapy for thyroid carcinoma. J Nucl Med 39:1551-1554
45. Mandel SJ, Mandel L (2003) Radioactive iodine and the salivary glands. Thyroid 13:265-271
46. Tsujii H (1985) Quantitative dose-response analysis of salivary function following radiotherapy using sequential RI-sialography. Int J Radiat Oncol Biol Phys 11:1603-1612
47. Van Acker F, Flamen P, Lambin P et al (2001) The utility of SPECT in determining the relationship between radiation dose and salivary gland dysfunction after radiotherapy. Nucl Med Commun. 22:225-231
48. Beal KP, Singh B, Kraus D et al (2003) Radiation-induced salivary gland tumors: a report of 18 cases and a review of the literature. Cancer J 9:467-471
49. Zhang L, Murata Y, Ishida R et al. Functional evaluation with intravoxel incoherent motion echo-planar MRI in irradiated salivary glands: a correlative study with salivary gland scintigraphy. J Magn Reson Imaging 14:223-229
50. Marks LB, Yu X, Vujaskovic Z et al (2003) Radiation-induced lung injury. Sem Radiat Oncol 13:333-345

Screening for Cardiovascular Disease in Survivors of Thoracic Radiation

M. Jacob Adams, Robert G. Prosnitz, Louis S. Constine, Lawrence B. Marks, and Steven E. Lipshultz

CONTENTS

7.1 Introduction 48
7.2 Methods 48
7.3 Types of Cardiovascular Complications 48
7.3.1 Overall Mortality from Cardiovascular Disease and Risk of Coronary Artery Disease 48
7.3.2 Cardiomyopathy 50
7.3.3 Valvular Disease 52
7.3.4 Conduction Abnormalities 52
7.3.5 Pericarditis 53
7.4 Indirect Effects on the Cardiovascular System 53
7.5 Screening and Diagnosis 54
7.6 Management 56
References 57

M. J. Adams, MD, MPH
Department of Community and Preventive Medicine, University of Rochester School of Medicine and Dentistry, P.O. Box 644, Rochester, NY 14642, USA
R. G. Prosnitz, MD, MPH
Department of Radiation Oncology, Duke University Medical Center, P.O. Box 3085, Durham, North Carolina 27710, USA
L. S. Constine, MD
Professor of Radiation Oncology and Pediatrics, Vice Chair, Department of Radiation Oncology, Departments of Radiation Oncology and Pediatrics, James P. Wilmot Cancer Center, University of Rochester Medical Center, P.O. Box 647 Rochester, NY 14642, USA
L. B. Marks MD
Professor, Department of Radiation Oncology, Duke University Medical Center, P.O. Box 3085, Durham, NC 27710, USA
S. E. Lipshultz, MD
Professor of Pediatrics, Medicine and Epidemiology and Public Health, Chair Department of Pediatrics, Associate Executive Dean for Child Health, Miller School of Medicine, University of Miami; Chief-of-Staff, Holtz Children's Hospital of the University of Miami-Jackson Memorial Medical Center; Director, Batchelor Children's Research Institute; Associate Director, Mailman Institute for Child Development; and Member, the Sylvester Comprehensive Cancer Center, University of Miami Miller School of Medicine, P.O. Box 016820, Miami, FL 33101, USA

Summary

Background and purpose: A solid body of evidence demonstrates that therapeutic thoracic radiotherapy can injure the cardiovascular system. However, there is little consensus on how to screen survivors who received this therapy. This review intends to assess recent evidence on radiotherapy-related cardiac injury with the goal of formulating evidence-based guidelines.

Material and methods: A literature search using Medline was performed in late 2004 to identify publications on the cardiovascular effects of thoracic radiation therapy (RT) that have been published since 2001. This search revealed 104 citations. After reviewing the abstracts, 40 were found to be irrelevant, and the remaining 59 articles and five comments on these articles were thoroughly reviewed.

Results: Recent publications confirmed the potential cardiotoxicity of thoracic radiotherapy in children and adults. These reports shed new light on radiation-associated cardiomyopathy and radiation-associated valvular disease, and they help to distinguish the cardiac effects of radiation in contrast to anthracyclines. The latest studies have also explored the use of new screening methodologies, though the prognostic significance of many of the abnormalities uncovered are presently unclear.

Conclusions: Although no screening protocol has been tested, recent evidence underscores the importance of comprehensive and repetitive cardiovascular screening of survivors treated with thoracic irradiation that incidentally exposed key cardiac structures to radiation.

7.1 Introduction

Over the last 40 years, overwhelming evidence has disproved the original assertion that the heart is radiation resistant. Despite this evidence, little consensus has developed about how to screen long-term cancer survivors treated with thoracic radiation. With a greater number of cancer patients surviving due to advances in multi-agent chemotherapy and radiotherapy, the need for evidence-based guidelines on how to screen these survivors becomes more critical. The primary purpose of this article is to discuss the recent literature on radiation-associated cardiovascular disease (CVD) and its implications for screening regimens of cancer survivors treated with thoracic radiation therapy (RT).

7.2 Methods

A literature search using Medline was performed to identify publications on the cardiovascular effects of RT that had been published since a similar review was written as a result of the last Late Effects of Normal Tissue Conference (LENT IV) [1]. The search strategy combined keyword searches of CVD, radiation, and Hodgkin's disease (HD) or breast cancer. Results were limited to English language articles and those published between 2001 and 2004. Focus was placed on HD and breast cancer because these are the most common cancers treated successfully with thoracic irradiation and thus there would be enough survivors to evaluate its long-term cardiotoxic effects. This search revealed 104 citations. More careful review of the citations suggested that 40 were not relevant or were not published in English, and five were letters to the editor regarding published articles. Of the remaining 59, 13 were large case series, case-control, or cohort studies (no intervention trials were uncovered), and were thus considered for inclusion into the study if they contributed new information to the field.

7.3 Types of Cardiovascular Complications

The potential adverse effects of thoracic radiation on the cardiovascular system are broad and are listed in Table 7.1. Historically, the most common adverse effect was pericarditis, but with modern RT doses and techniques the most common and feared adverse effect is the increased risk of fatal myocardial infarction. Table 7.3 lists those factors that increase the risk of suffering a radiation-associated cardiac complication.

7.3.1 Overall Mortality from Cardiovascular Disease and Risk of Coronary Artery Disease

Multiple studies have demonstrated that HD survivors treated with mediastinal irradiation are at increased risk of fatal CVD [2–7]. Relative risk estimates for survivors generally range between 2.2 and 7.2, compared to the age- and gender- matched general population [2–7]. Absolute excess risk of fatal CVD ranges from 11.9 to 48.9 per 10,000 patient years depending upon patient characteristics [4]. This increased risk becomes statistically significant 5–10 years after radiotherapy, and is largely due to fatal myocardial infarctions (MI) [4, 6]. Survivors of childhood HD treated with older techniques of RT appear to be at even higher relative risk [5, 8]. A retrospective study from Stanford demonstrated that HD survivors treated at <21 years of age between 1961 and 1991 suffered fatal MI 41.5 times more often than the age-matched general population [5]. Deaths occurred 3–22 years after therapy. These deaths were limited to those exposed to ≥42 Gy of radiation. A total of 71% of this cohort received ≥40 Gy. Although it is uncommon to treat children today with doses >30 Gy, it is unclear whether limiting exposure has impacted the rate of fatal MI in HD survivors [7].

Women treated with older methods of adjuvant irradiation after mastectomy for left-sided breast cancer have been shown to have an increased incidence of fatal CVD [9–14]. Concern was raised by post-hoc analyses showing that women who received adjuvant RT had a higher rate of cardiac death than unirradiated patients [9, 10, 15]. Tumor registry studies comparing cardiovascular-related mortality in women

Table 7.1. Spectrum of radiation-induced cardiovascular disease. (Modified from [80] with permission)

Manifestation	Comments
Pericarditis	1. During therapy – Associated with mediastinal tumor and some chemotherapy agents such as cyclophosphamide [76] 2. Post-therapy – Acute effusion, chronic effusion, pericarditis, constrictive pericarditis. Seen with high doses of RT and large volumes of heart within the RT field [76]
Myocardial fibrosis	1. Fibrosis secondary to microvasculature changes [76] 2. Frequently with normal left ventricular dimensions, ejection fraction and fractional shortening as measured by radionuclide scan or echocardiogram [77] 3. Progressive, restrictive cardiomyopathy with fibrosis may occur. This can lead to pulmonary vascular disease and pulmonary hypertension [77] 4. Diastolic dysfunction may occur alone as well as with systolic dysfunction [77]
Coronary artery disease	1. The structural changes in the coronary arteries associated with radiation therapy are essentially the same as those of ordinary atherosclerosis [76] 2. Premature fibrosis may accelerate atherosclerosis [78, 79] 3. Distribution of arteries affected tends to be anterior with anterior weighted RT [76] 4. Lesions tend to be proximal and even ostial [78, 79] 5. ↑ Rates of silent ischemia (see autonomic effects) [54]
Valvular disease	1. Predominantly mitral valve and aortic valve [47] 2. ↑ Regurgitation and stenosis with ↑ time since therapy [47]
Conduction system/ arrhythmia	1. Complete or incomplete right bundle branch block is suggestive of right bundle branch fibrosis [51] 2. Initial conduction abnormalities may progress to complete heart block and cause congestive heart failure, requiring a pacemaker [51] 3. Complete heart block rarely occurs without other radiation-associated abnormalities of the heart [51]
Autonomic dysfunction	1. Frequent cardiac dysfunction with tachycardia, loss of circadian rhythm and respiratory phasic heart rate variability [54] 2. Signs listed in #1 are similar to a denervated heart. This raises the question of whether such changes in survivors are related to autonomic nervous system damage [54] 3. ↓ Perception of anginal pain [54]

with left-sided vs. right-sided breast cancer raised similar concerns about the cardiotoxicity of RT for breast cancer [13, 14]. Relative risk estimates of fatal MI after left-sided RT range as high as 2.2 compared with women who were treated for right-sided breast cancer [14]. Further evaluation has revealed that the increased risk appears limited to those who received the highest dose-volumes of cardiac radiation (women with left-sided malignancy whose irradiation fields included the internal mammary nodes) [12, 16].

To our knowledge, only one study has evaluated coronary heart disease clinical events in breast cancer survivors treated solely with modern techniques after mastectomy. This randomized trial of post-mastectomy RT by Hojris et al. [17] did not show a significant difference in ischemic heart disease mortality or morbidity from breast irradiation at a median follow-up of 10 years. Although the RT treated and non-treated groups were not perfectly balanced in terms of laterality of breast cancer, a sub-analysis in only the patients with left-sided breast cancer revealed no increased risk of ischemic heart disease or acute myocardial infarction incidence. However, the shorter median follow-up in this study, compared with the studies looking at older techniques of RT, may not have provided enough time to observe a sufficient number of cardiac events attributable to RT (i.e., excess events over the baseline high rate in Western societies). This problem is compounded by the fact that one would expect a slower rate of events, because modern techniques decrease the heart's dose-volume of exposure. Thus more time would be required to see the same absolute adverse effect.

Studies using clinical imaging of the heart underscore the danger of prematurely concluding that the newer methods of RT pose no risk to the heart. Investigators from several institutions have evaluated the heart in patients treated for breast cancer with cardiac perfusion imaging. Researchers at Duke University have accumulated the largest series of patients. Between 1998 and 2001, 114 patients with left-sided breast cancer underwent pre- and serial post-RT single photon emission computed tomography (SPECT) gated cardiac perfusion scans. Studies published on this cohort of patients demonstrate that: (1) RT to the left chest wall/breast using modern techniques causes perfusion defects in 50%–63% of women 6–24 months post-RT [18]; (2) that the incidence of perfusion defects is associated with the volume of left ventricle irradiated; [3] that the perfusion defects generally persist 3–5 years post-RT [19]; and (4) that the perfusion defects are associated with abnormalities in regional wall motion [20], subtle reductions in ejection fraction [20], and episodes of chest pain [21]. These findings are consistent with other smaller series [22–25]. Lind suggested that the incidence of such perfusion defects was associated with pre-treatment serum cholesterol [26]. The risk of fatal CVD associated with adjuvant radiotherapy after breast-conserving surgery (BCS) appears to be much less than the risk following post-mastectomy RT (PMRT) [27]. The risk following RT after BCS may be lower because, in contrast to PMRT, a substantial proportion of patients treated following BCS do not receive regional node radiation. The chief indication for PMRT is involved axillary lymph nodes. Thus, the regional nodes are almost always irradiated in patients treated after mastectomy. In contrast, many patients irradiated following BCS do not have axillary node metastases. In these patients, only the breast is irradiated. (The breast and regional nodes are generally irradiated following BCS in node-positive patients.) When the regional nodes are not treated, the volume of heart incidentally irradiated is typically reduced. Whether any increased risk is associated with adjuvant RT after BCS has been the subject of three studies comparing patients treated in this setting by laterality of the cancer [28–30]. Only one revealed an increased risk, and it was minimal [29]. This population-based cohort study of patients treated between 1982 and 1987 in Ontario, Canada, demonstrated that the 1555 women with left-sided cancer had a 2.1 greater risk (after age adjustment) of fatal MI than the 1451 with right-sided malignancy, 8–14 years after diagnosis. Absolute incidence was 2% versus 1%, respectively [29]. The minimal absolute difference may be explained by the fact that ≤5% of the left ventricle is generally exposed to radiation after breast conserving therapy.

The overall pattern of risk in the three survivor populations (HD, breast cancer treated with RT after mastectomy, and breast cancer treated with RT after lumpectomy) highlights the importance of radiation dose and the volume of exposure to the heart in determining the risk of future adverse cardiovascular events.

7.3.2
Cardiomyopathy

The nature of cardiac dysfunction seen following RT may differ in patients treated with RT alone compared with patients who also received potentially cardiotoxic chemotherapy (e.g., anthracyclines). Because radiation causes fibrosis of the myocardium, restrictive cardiomyopathy (Fig. 7.1), characterized by diastolic dysfunction, predominates in survivors treated with RT alone. In contrast, systolic dysfunction usually dominates in survivors who also received anthracyclines [31]. Although clinically evident heart failure is rare in survivors treated with radiotherapy alone, studies evaluating survivors with imaging technologies show that subclinical changes are common and may be progressive. The concern is that these subclinical diastolic abnormalities may progress over the long-term to systolic dysfunction, congestive heart failure or both.

One of the earliest studies using cardiac function imaging technology evaluated 21 asymptomatic adult survivors of HD treated prior to 1983 with 20–76 Gy (mean 35.9 Gy) of mediastinal RT without chemotherapy. In this case series, 57% had an abnormal left and/or right ventricular ejection fraction, 7–20 years after treatment (mean 14.1 years) [32]. Constine et al. evaluated 50 HD survivors who had been treated with modern radiotherapy techniques to 18.5–47.5 Gy (mean 35.1 Gy) up to 30 years previously (mean 9.1 years) [33]. On evaluation with radionuclide ventriculography, 4% had an abnormal left ventricular ejection fraction, and 16% had an abnormal peak filling rate, an indirect measure of diastolic function. Adams et al. reported findings that suggest a greater impact from diastolic dysfunction than from systolic abnormalities, after radiotherapy alone [34]. This investigation comprehensively evaluated cardiac status in 48 long-term survivors of childhood or young adolescent HD treated with mantle irradiation (range, 27.0–51.7 Gy; median, 40 Gy). Only four patients had received anthracyclines. At a median 14.3 years after diagnosis, 12%

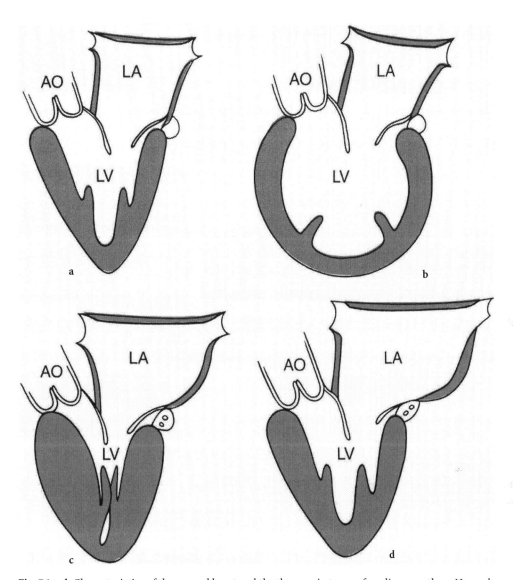

Fig. 7.1a–d. Characteristics of the normal heart and the three main types of cardiomyopathy. a Normal. b Dilated cardiomyopathy: Note the thin left ventricular (*LV*) walls and enlarged LV chamber, resulting in poor contraction of heart muscle (systolic dysfunction). c Hypertrophic cardiomyopathy: not related to the cardiotoxicity of cancer therapy. d Restrictive cardiomyopathy: note the normal to slightly thickened LV walls and slightly decreased LV chamber size. These changes are caused by fibrosis which stiffens the myocardium and results in poor chamber filling (diastolic dysfunction). (Reproduced from [75] with permission)

had an abnormal measure of systolic function, but three of these five patients had received an anthracycline as well. In contrast, 37.2% had an abnormal measure of LV mass and/or end diastolic dimension. Both reduced LV mass and reduced end diastolic dimension are suggestive of restrictive cardiomyopathy. In addition, the E/A ratio (a measure of peak early filling to peak late filling of the left ventricle that serves as a screening measurement for diastolic dysfunction) was measured in 37 patients. Twelve (32%) had probable abnormal E/A ratios between 1.5 and 2.0, and 8 (22%) had a definite abnormal ratio ≥2.0. These studies demonstrate that the type and prevalence of dysfunction varies depending upon treatment, length of follow-up, and method of screening. They also illustrate that radiation-associated cardiomyopathy is more likely to be restrictive in nature and thus affect diastolic function rather than systolic, though systolic function can also be impacted with very high radiation doses and long follow-up.

Many survivors of HD and breast cancer have received both thoracic radiation and anthracyclines. As early as the 1970s, reports [35–37] suggested that radiation to the heart in conjunction with anthracyclines is associated with greater cardiac toxicity than either modality in isolation [38]. Radiation injures the endothelium of myocardial capillaries leading to ischemia and ultimately myocardial fibrosis. Doxorubicin principally damages myocytes directly; its ultimate result is primarily systolic dysfunction. Studies evaluating long-term survivors of childhood cancer [39], young adulthood HD [34, 40] and breast cancer [41] have confirmed that combined therapy affects cardiac morbidity and mortality more significantly than either alone.

7.3.3
Valvular Disease

Prospective studies of HD survivors treated with ≥30 Gy of mediastinal RT, published before 2000, report a frequency of pathologic (greater than grade 1) left-sided valvular regurgitation ranging between 16%–40% [42–45]. Only in the largest (n = 116) was a comparison with a control group provided. In this study by Lund et al., which screened 90% of the eligible HD survivors treated between 1980 and 1988 with RT techniques no longer in use, 31% of patients had pathologic left-sided regurgitation 5–13 years after therapy [45]. No pathological left-sided regurgitation was observed in the comparison group of 40 healthy volunteers. However, it was not clear how well the control group matched the survivors.

Two recent studies have compared the prevalence of valvular abnormalities in HD survivors treated with RT versus the frequency in age- and gender-matched controls from the general population based on data from the Framingham Heart Study. In the series by Adams et al. (previously discussed) in which comprehensive cardiac screening was performed in 48 survivors of HD treated with mediastinal RT, 42.6% had at least one significant valve abnormality [34]. Heidenreich et al. have performed the largest study to date of 294 asymptomatic HD survivors treated 2 to >20 years previously [46]. They demonstrated that survivors treated with a mean mantle dose of 43 Gy had a several-fold increased risk of any significant valvular disease compared with the general population of a similar age. The most striking increase was the 34-fold higher risk of aortic regurgitation >grade 2 (an absolute incidence of 26.1%) [46]. This study also illustrated that the frequency of significant aortic regurgitation, aortic stenosis, and mitral regurgitation each increased with longer follow-up. Although a decrease in the radiation exposure to the heart likely occurred as techniques improved, this finding adds to the significant previous data suggesting that radiation-associated valvular disease is progressive [1, 47].

In summary, valvular insufficiency is more frequent than stenosis, but the latter more often has hemodynamic significance requiring intervention [47]. These studies also suggest that a threshold dose for valvular regurgitation exists at approximately 30 Gy of mediastinal radiation when patients are evaluated 15 years after therapy. In terms of clinical significance, many of the valvular abnormalities that have been reported would lead to recommendations for endocarditis prophylaxis. In fact, Heidenreich et al. report that patients in their study who had survived ≥10 years, only four survivors would need to be screened to uncover one who would be eligible for endocarditis prophylaxis [46]. Furthermore, a recent study by Hull et al. indicates an eight-fold increase in the risk of valve repair surgeries in HD survivors compared with the general population [48].

Only one uncontrolled study has evaluated valvular disease in breast cancer survivors. The frequency and severity of valvular abnormalities was low and probably no different than in untreated women of the same age [49]. The risk of radiation-associated valvular disease in breast cancer survivors requires additional investigation, although the risk is probably much less than in HD patients treated with RT.

7.3.4
Conduction Abnormalities

Radiation may cause fibrosis of the conduction pathways of the cardiac system, potentially leading to life threatening arrhythmias and/or conduction defects years after therapy. Numerous case reports and case series have demonstrated the various conduction abnormalities and conduction defects associated with mediastinal RT, including atrioventricular nodal bradycardia, all levels of heart block, including complete heart block [50, 51] and sick sinus syndrome [51, 52]. These are different from the frequent, asymptomatic, nonspecific, and transient repolarization abnormalities seen shortly after irradiation [53].

Few prospective studies, however, have looked at the frequency of conduction defects in long-term survivors. In a study of 134 childhood cancer survivors at a mean of 5 years after treatment with anthracyclines and/or mediastinal irradiation, ventricular tachycardia was significantly greater in those treated with chest RT, irrespective of anthracycline treatment, than in a group of historical controls [53]. The frequency of prolonged QT interval was 12.5% in those treated with chest irradiation alone, 11% in those treated with anthracycline alone, and 18.9% in those treated with both. In the comprehensive cardiac screening study performed by Adams et al., 74.5% of the HD survivors treated with mediastinal radiotherapy had a conduction defect or arrhythmia [34]. An RSR prime pattern in the right precordial leads was the most common defect, occurring in >50% of survivors; it indicates a conduction delay in the right anterior bundle, the most anterior structure of the intracardiac conduction system. Two other survivors had complete right-bundle-branch block. These results suggest that the most anterior structures of the intracardiac conduction system are most at risk for fibrosis from mediastinal RT.

Results of 24-h electrocardiogram from the Adams et al. study suggested a high rate of autonomic dysfunction, with 31% of survivors having sustained tachycardia and 57% having a monotonous heart rate [34]. A concern is that autonomic nervous system dysfunction could lead to the decreased perception of anginal chest pain, and this has been reported in some HD survivors previously treated with mediastinal RT [54].

The frequency of serious conduction abnormalities in survivors of adult cancer treated with chest irradiation appears to be low. A study of 69 breast cancer survivors treated with adjuvant radiotherapy found the incidence of conduction/rhythm abnormalities to be increased above baseline at 6 months and at 10 years post-treatment [55]. Although changes occurred more often in those with left-sided malignancy, none of the abnormalities compromised function, nor was the frequency of ischemic changes on exercise stress testing different from the expected rate in healthy women of the same age.

Symptoms from conduction abnormalities range from palpitations to syncope to sudden death, but are uncommon. Conduction defects, which produce symptoms, rarely occur without some other radiation-induced cardiac injury [50].

7.3.5
Pericarditis

Although pericarditis was historically one of the most common cardiac complications of mediastinal irradiation, it rarely occurs after the modern techniques and lower total doses used currently. At one center, the incidence of pericarditis decreased from 20% to 2.5% with changes in methods of RT in the 1970s [56]. Signs and symptoms of pericarditis are the same as in the general population.

7.4
Indirect Effects on the Cardiovascular System

Depending on dosage and targeting, thoracic RT can affect other structures in the neck and chest, which the heart depends upon to function properly (Table 7.2). Radiation-associated fibrosis of the lungs, skeletal muscle damage, and scoliosis due to radiation can affect cardiopulmonary function [1]. One study of 92 HD survivors treated with RT +/− chemotherapy from 1980 to 1988 demonstrated that those with pulmonary function testing abnormalities were three times more likely to report fatigue on a standardized instrument than those without abnormalities [57]. Radiation can cause stenosis and fibrosis of the carotid arteries, the aorta, and the branch pulmonary arteries [58]. Clinical presentations include transient ischemic attacks, stroke, carotid bruit, vertebrobasilar insufficiency, and upper- or lower-

Table 7.2. Indirect effects of mediastinal radiation on the cardiovascular system. (Modified from [80] with permission)

Manifestation	Comments
Mediastinal fibrosis	↓ Success of cardiovascular surgery [71]
Lung fibrosis	Chronic, restrictive and can be progressive [60]
Scoliosis and ↓ skeletal muscle	↓ Cardiovascular and lung function [60]
Thyroid	Usually hypothyroid [81] Affects cardiovascular function and lipid profile. May cause pericarditis
Thoracic duct fibrosis	Chylothorax-late onset and extremely rare [59]

extremity insufficiency. The very rare diagnosis of a chylothorax due to thoracic duct fibrosis should be considered in patients with symptoms of late onset heart failure and unexplained pericardial effusion [59]. Thyroid dysfunction after mantle irradiation is common and can occur anytime after therapy [60]. Hypothyroidism may lead to obesity and dyslipidemia, both risk factors for coronary heart disease. Hypothyroidism can also cause decreased ventricular contractility, ventricular diastolic dysfunction, arrhythmias, congestive heart failure, and chronic pericardial effusion that can lead to symptoms and, rarely, tamponade [60]. Early recognition and treatment of subclinical hypothyroidism is key because, once cardiovascular dysfunction occurs, it may not resolve even after the patient's hypothyroidism is treated appropriately.

7.5 Screening and Diagnosis

Although no screening regimens have been rigorously tested, the recent literature reinforces the notion that screening should involve multiple testing modalities and occur repeatedly over time (Table 7.4)
[61]. Serial screening is needed because the course of cardiac disease progression is unknown but is probably progressive and may vary between individuals. In addition, early detection and appropriate treatment of cardiac abnormalities may prevent or minimize morbidity and mortality. Screening is also performed more frequently in children because the irradiated heart may not have a normal hypertrophic response to keep pace with the demands of a growing body. For a similar reason, women who received mediastinal radiotherapy ought to be referred to a cardiologist at the time (or contemplation) of pregnancy for serial screening throughout pregnancy [62].

The wide range of possible cardiac abnormalities associated with thoracic RT suggests the potential usefulness of multiple screening modalities (Table 7.3). Those at highest risk for cardiovascular abnormalities are childhood cancer survivors, HD survivors treated with outdated techniques exposing large volumes of the heart to ≥35 Gy, and survivors treated with an anthracycline. These survivors, as well as others with characteristics that suggest higher risk (Table 7.4), should be screened regularly for myocardial dysfunction and coronary heart disease. Other survivors treated with chest radiotherapy may also benefit from increased attention.

Table 7.3. Risk factors for the different manifestations of radiation-induced heart disease. (Modified from [80] with permission)

Risk factor	Pericarditis	CM	CAD	Arrhythmia	Valvular disease	All causes CD
Total dose: (>30–35 Gy) [47, 76, 82]	X	X	X	X	X	X
Fraction Size: (≥2.0 Gy/day) [76]	X	X	X	Likely	Likely	X
Volume of heart exposed [76]	X	X	X	Likely	Likely	X
Anterior weighting of AP/PA radiation fields [4, 76]	X	X	X	Likely	Likely	X
Tumor adjacent to heart [76]	X	–	–	–	–	–
Younger age at exposure [5, 76, 83]	–	X	X	Likely	Likely	X
Increased time since exposure (latency) [4, 46, 47, 51, 84]	–	X	X	X	X	X
Type of radiation source [76]	X	X	X	Likely	Likely	X
Use of adjuvant cardiotoxic chemotherapy [76, 85]	–	X	–	X	X	X
Co-existing classical CHD risk factors [76, 82]	–	–	X	–	–	X

CM, cardiomyopathy; *CAD*, coronary artery disease; *CD*, cardiac death; –, no known association; *Likely*, unknown but likely association; *X*, associations of specific risk factors with specific presentation.

Table 7.4. Evaluation and treatment of patients at risk for late effects of thoracic radiotherapy. (Modified from [60] with permission)

Late effects	Treatment[a]	Signs and symptoms	Screening and diagnostic tests	Management and intervention
Pericarditis	>35 Gy	Fatigue, dyspnea on exertion, chest pain, cyanosis, ascites, peripheral edema, hypotension, friction rub, muffled heart sounds, venous distension, pulses paradoxus, Kussmaul's sign	Electrocardiogram Chest X-ray Echocardiogram	Pericardiocentesis Pericardiectomy
Cardiomyopathy (myocardial disease)	>35 Gy or >25 Gy and anthracycline	Fatigue, cough, dyspnea on exertion, peripheral edema, hypertension, tachypnea, rales, tachycardia, murmur, extra heart sounds, hepatomegaly, syncope, palpitations	Echocardiogram and/or radionuclide ventriculography – Evaluate diastolic and systolic function	Education regarding risks of: alcohol, isometric exercise, smoking and other drug use, pregnancy, and anesthesia Afterload reducers, beta-blocker, antiarrhythmics, diuretics, digoxin Cardiac transplant
Coronary heart disease	>30 Gy	Chest pain, dyspnea, diaphoresis, hypotension, pallor, nausea, arrhythmia	Exercise or dobutamine stress test with radionuclide perfusion imaging, or echocardiography (frequency depends on risk factor profile and symptoms)	Risk factor modifications including diet and conditioning regimens Cardiac medications and lipid lowering agents Coronary artery bypass graft or angioplasty
Valvular disease	>30 Gy	Cough, weakness, dyspnea on exertion, new murmur, rales, peripheral edema or any other sign of congestive heart failure	Echocardiogram Cardiac catheterization	Ampicillin prophylaxis for dental or surgical procedures Replacement of valve
Arrhythmia		Palpitations, light-headedness, syncope	Electrocardiogram and 24-h ECG Evaluation for other abnormalities	Pacemaker

[a] Cumulative radiation exposure of the mediastinum at this level or higher clearly indicates increased risk for the specific complication and thus the need to screen for it; however, the complication may also occur at lower doses.

All survivors of cancer treated with thoracic radiotherapy should be monitored on an ongoing basis for coronary heart disease risk factors such as obesity, hypertension, dyslipidemias, and diabetes because of the large public health burden of coronary heart disease and the availability of effective preventive measures. Screening should start soon after completion of therapy regardless of the patient's age, given that fatal myocardial infarctions have even occurred in survivors during childhood. Screening should continue throughout the patient's life, since the deleterious effects of incidental cardiac irradiation may not manifest for many years. The revised National Cholesterol Education Panel recommendations provide a well thought out minimum of care that should be provided for the screening and treatment of dyslipidemias [63]. Radiation exposure should be counted as a risk factor, along with those listed in the guidelines, in determining the LDL-cholesterol goal of therapy. Children and women of childbearing potential with abnormal lipid levels should be referred to a specialist who regularly treats such patients because the teratogenicity and the long-term safety of the most commonly used drugs have not been well studied in children. All survivors should be educated about the cardiotoxic risks of their treatments, and, when appropriate, about the need for lifelong monitoring of heart function.

Serial echocardiography and radionuclide ventriculography, also called radionuclide angiography, are useful for following myocardial function. Both are reliable methods of measuring left ventricular systolic performance. Echocardiography is non-invasive and is able to assess the anatomic structures of the heart such as the pericardium, and ventricular walls and valves. Diastolic function can and should be indirectly measured by Doppler echocardiography. Unfortunately, echocardiography is of poor quality in many adults because of body habitus and bone density. Radionuclide imaging may therefore be necessary for repeated quantitative analysis of systolic function in certain patients. However, diastolic function is difficult to measure with the radionuclide technology found in many hospitals. This is of particular concern in those treated with thoracic RT because diastolic dysfunction is more likely to occur than systolic dysfunction. It should also be noted that the ejection fraction measured with echocardiography and the ejection fraction on RNA are not directly convertible [64]. Myocardial function should therefore be assessed with echocardiography with or without radionuclide studies, depending on the quality of the former in a particular patient.

Exercise or pharmacologic (e.g., dobutamine) stress testing augments the diagnosis of ischemic heart disease and cardiac dysfunction compared with rest-only studies. Radionuclide myocardial perfusion scanning during exercise has 90% sensitivity and specificity in the general population to detect ischemic heart disease. However, the sensitivity and specificity of this test in irradiated patients has not been well studied. Radionuclide myocardial perfusion scanning appears to detect radiation-induced microvascular damage in the myocardium [18, 65], but the ability of perfusion scanning to distinguish microvascular abnormalities from coronary heart disease in this population is unclear. However, the detection of microvascular damage may identify those who are at highest risk for heart failure and death, although this requires further study [20, 21].

Maximal oxygen consumption, a variable that can be measured during exercise stress testing, has been shown to have prognostic significance in patients with cardiomyopathy [66]. Reports by Adams and others have documented that maximal oxygen consumption is surprisingly low in many patients with prior mediastinal irradiation, including those who did not have symptoms of cardiac dysfunction [34, 39]. Adams et al. also found that of all the measures of cardiac status analyzed, maximal oxygen consumption was the only one to be highly correlated with the physical component of quality of life on the SF36 [34]. Pulmonary function tests were not performed, so it is unclear to what extent pulmonary dysfunction, which has been shown to be correlated with quality of life in HD survivors treated with mediastinal RT [57], caused decreased maximal oxygen consumption.

Although screening for electrical conduction abnormalities and rhythm disturbances may in theory be reasonable because they can remain silent until fatal, it is not clear that these abnormalities occur frequently enough to warrant screening all survivors who received mediastinal RT. Furthermore, the prognostic value of the various non-specific conduction abnormalities observed in this population remains unknown. Nevertheless, there is clear value in repeatedly screening survivors with congestive heart failure. In these patients, a 24-h ECG can detect silent arrhythmia that could be treated with a pacemaker and thus reduce mortality [67]. Invasive procedures are not necessary for screening purposes. Cardiac catheterization and angiography are appropriate, however, for diagnostic purposes to evaluate heart failure and angina.

7.6
Management

The treatment of radiation-associated CVD differs little from the procedures used in the general population with the same disease. Unfortunately, much less is known about the treatment of heart failure due to the diastolic dysfunction associated with restrictive cardiomyopathy than the more common systolic dysfunction seen with dilated cardiomyopathy. Careful, early, invasive assessment of hemodynamics, followed by aggressive, tailored, pharmacologic therapy and early heart transplantation has been beneficial [68]. However, before transplantation is considered, all reversible factors should be treated and the medical regimen should be optimized. Surgical interventions for coronary heart disease and valvular disease are generally successful in irradiated patients unless extensive mediastinal fibrosis is present (primarily a concern in patients treated to high RT doses or using large doses per fraction). Thus, there are multiple extra precautions that should be considered when performing surgery in the survivor treated with thoracic irradiation [69–74].

In conclusion, radiotherapy that includes the heart in the treatment field can lead to a broad range of cardiac complications, many of which appear to be progressive. Over the last few years our appreciation of the cardiovascular late effects of thoracic RT has grown, particularly in demonstrating the prevalence of significant valvular defects in survivors and early evidence demonstrating widespread perfusion defects in such patients. The prevalence of these cardiac abnormalities has strengthened the case for periodic screening with multiple testing modalities. Although radiation-induced heart disease is treated similarly to heart disease in the general population, special precautions should be taken because of the changes radiation causes to the heart and other structures in the chest.

Acknowledgements

This work was supported by the National Institutes of Health (CA-79060, HL-070830), the Wilmot Cancer Research Fellowship of the James P. Wilmot Foundation, and the Department of Defense (BC010663 and DAMD 179818071).

References

1. Adams MJ, Lipshultz SE, Schwartz C (2003) Radiation-associated cardiovascular disease: manifestations and management. Semin Radiat Oncol 13:346–356
2. Lee CK, Aeppli D, Nierengarten ME (2000) The need for long-term surveillance for patients treated with curative radiotherapy for Hodgkin's disease: University of Minnesota experience. Int J Radiat Oncol Biol Phys 48:169–179
3. Mauch P, Kalish LA, Marcus KC (1995) Long-term survival in Hodgkin's disease: relative impact of mortality, second tumors, infection and cardiovascular disease. Cancer J Scientific Am 1:33–42
4. Hancock SL, Tucker MA, Hoppe RT (1993) Factors affecting late mortality from heart disease after treatment for Hodgkin's disease. JAMA 270:1949–1955
5. Hancock SL, Donaldson SS, Hoppe RT (1993) Cardiac disease following treatment of Hodgkin's disease in children and adolescents. J Clin Oncol 11:1208–1215
6. Reinders JG, Heijmen BJ, Olofsen-van Acht MJ (1999) Ischemic heart disease after mantlefield irradiation for Hodgkin's disease in long-term follow-up. Radiother Oncol 51:35–42
7. Boivin J-F, Hutchison G, Lubin J (1992) Coronary artery disease mortality in patients treated for Hodgkin's disease. Cancer 69:1241–1247
8. Aleman BM, van den Belt-Dusebout AW, Klokman WJ (2003) Long-term cause-specific mortality of patients treated for Hodgkin's disease. J Clin Oncol 21:3431–3439
9. Jones JM, Ribeiro GG (1989) Mortality pattern over 34 years of breast cancer patients in a clinical trial of post-operative radiotherapy. Clin Radiol 40:204–208
10. Cuzick J, Stewart H, Rutqvist L (1994) Cause-specific mortality in long-term survivors of breast cancer who participated in trials of radiotherapy. J Clin Oncol 12:447–453
11. Early Breast Cancer Trialists' Collaborative Group (1990) Treatment of early breast cancer, vol. 1, worldwide evidence, 1985–1990. Oxford University, Oxford
12. Rutqvist LE, Lax I, Fornander T (1992) Cardiovascular mortality in a randomized trial of adjuvant radiation therapy versus surgery alone in primary breast cancer. Int J Radiat Oncol Biol Phys 22:887–896
13. Rutqvist LE, Johansson H (1990) Mortality by laterality of the primary tumor among 55,000 breast cancer patients from the Swedish center registry. Br J Cancer 61:866–868
14. Paszat LF, Mackillop WJ, Groome PA (1998) Mortality from myocardial infarction after adjuvant radiotherapy for breast cancer in the surveillance, epidemiology, and end-results cancer registries. J Clin Oncol 16:2625–2631
15. Cuzick J, Stewart H, Peto R (1987) Overview of randomized trials of postoperative adjuvant radiotherapy in breast cancer. Cancer Treat Reports 71:15–29
16. Gyenes G, Rutqvist LE, Liedberg A (1998) Long-term cardiac morbidity and mortality in a randomized trial of pre- and post-operative radiation therapy versus surgery alone in primary breast cancer. Radiother Oncol 48:185–190
17. Hojris I, Overgaard M, Christensen JJ (1999) Morbidity and mortality of ischaemic heart disease in high-risk breast-cancer patients after adjuvant postmastectomy systemic treatment with or without radiotherapy: analysis of DBCG 82b and 82c randomized trials. Radiotherapy Committee of the Danish Breast Cancer Cooperative Group. Lancet 354:1425–1430
18. Hardenbergh PH, Munley MT, Bentel GC (2001) Cardiac perfusion changes in patients treated for breast cancer with radiation therapy and doxorubicin: preliminary results. Int J Radiat Oncol Biol Phys 49:1023–1028
19. Yu X, Zhou S, Kahn D (2004) Persistence of radiation (RT)-induced cardiac perfusion defects 3–5 years post RT (abstract). J Clin Oncol (Meeting Abstracts) 22:33b
20. Marks LB, Prosnitz RG, Hardenberg PH (2002) Functional consequences of radiation (RT)-induced perfusion changes in patients with left-sided breast cancer. Program and abstracts of the American Society for Therapeutic Radiology and Oncology 44th Annual Meeting; October 6–10; New Orleans, Louisiana. Abstract 1
21. Yu X, Prosnitz RR, Zhou S (2003) Symptomatic cardiac events following radiation therapy for left-sided breast cancer: possible association with radiation therapy-induced changes in regional perfusion. Clin Breast Cancer 4:193–197
22. Gyenes G, Fornander T, Carlens P (1994) Morbidity of ischemic heart disease in early breast cancer 15–20 years after adjuvant radiotherapy. Int J Radiat Oncol Biol Phys 28:1235–1241

23. Cowen D, Gonzague-Casabianca L, Brenot-Rossi I (1907) Thallium-201 perfusion scintigraphy in the evaluation of late myocardial damage in left-sided breast cancer. Int J Radiat Oncol Biol Phys 41:809–815
24. Hojris I, Sand NP, Andersen J (2000) Myocardial perfusion imaging in breast cancer patients treated with or without post-mastectomy radiotherapy. Radiother Oncol 55:163–172
25. Seddon B, Cook A, Gothard L (2002) Detection of defects in myocardial perfusion imaging in patients with early breast cancer treated with radiotherapy. Radiother Oncol 64:53–63
26. Lind PA, Pagnanelli R, Marks LB (2003) Myocardial perfusion changes in patients irradiated for left-sided breast cancer and correlation with coronary artery distribution. Int J Radiat Oncol Biol Phys 55:914–920
27. Rutqvist LE, Liedberg A, Hammar N (1998) Myocardial infarction among women with early-stage breast cancer treated with conservative surgery and breast irradiation. Int J Radiat Oncol Biol Phys 40:359–363
28. Nixon AJ, Manola J, Gelman R (1998) No long term increase in cardiac related mortality after breast-conserving surgery and radiation therapy using modern techniques. J Clin Oncol 16:1374–1379
29. Paszat LF, Mackillop WJ, Groome PA (1999) Mortality from myocardial infarction following postlumpectomy radiotherapy for breast cancer: population-based study in Ontario, Canada. Int J Radiat Oncol Biol Phys 43:755–762
30. Vallis KA, Pintilie M, Chong N (2002) Assessment of coronary heart disease morbidity and mortality after radiation therapy for early breast cancer. J Clin Oncol 20:1036–1042
31. Tolba KA, Deliargyris EN (1999) Cardiotoxicity of cancer therapy. Cancer Invest 17:408–422
32. Burns RJ, Bar Shlomo BZ, Druck MN (1983) Detection of radiation cardiomyopathy by gated radionuclide angiography. Am J Med 74:297–301
33. Constine LS, Schwartz RG, Savage D (1997) Cardiac function, perfusion, and morbidity in irradiated long-term survivors of Hodgkin's disease. Int J Radiat Oncol Biol Phys 39:897–906
34. Adams MJ, Lipsitz SR, Colan SD (2004) Cardiovascular status in long-term survivors of Hodgkin's disease treated with chest radiotherapy. J Clin Oncol 22:3139–3148
35. Billingham ME, Bristow MR, Glatstein E (1977) Adriamycin cardiotoxicity: endomyocardial biopsy evidence of enhancement by irradiation. Am J Surg Pathol 1:17–23
36. Merrill J, Geco FA, Zimber H (1975) Adriamycin and radiation: synergistic cardiotoxicity (abstract). Ann Intern Med 82:122–123
37. Kinsella TJ, Ahmann DL, Giuliani ER (1979) Adriamycin toxicity in stage IV breast cancer: possible enhancement with prior left chest radiation therapy. Int J Radiat Oncol Biol Phys 5:1979–2002
38. Fajardo LF, Eltringham JR, Stewart JR (1976) Combined cardiotoxicity of adriamycin and x-radiation. Lab Invest 34:86–96
39. Pihkala J, Happonen JM, Virtanen K (1995) Cardiopulmonary evaluation of exercise tolerance after chest irradiation and anticancer chemotherapy in children and adolescents. Pediatrics 95:722–726
40. Leonard GT, Green DM, Spangenthal EL (2000) Cardiac mortality and morbidity after treatment for Hodgkin disease during childhood and adolescence (abstract). Pediatr Res 47:46A
41. Shapiro CL, Hardenbergh PH, Gelman R (1998) Cardiac effects of adjuvant doxorubicin and radiation therapy in breast cancer patients. J Clin Oncol 16:3493–3501
42. Glanzmann C, Huguenin P, Lutolf UM (1994) Cardiac lesions after mediastinal radiation for Hodgkin's disease. Radiother Oncol 30:43–54
43. Kreuser ED, Voller H, Behles C (1993) Evaluation of late cardiotoxicity with pulsed Doppler echocardiography in patients treated for Hodgkin's disease. Br J Haematol 84:615–622
44. Gustavsson A, Eskilsson J, Landberg T (1990) Late cardiac effects after mantle radiation in patients with Hodgkin's disease. Ann Oncol 1:355–363
45. Lund MB, Ihlen H, Voss BM (1996) Increased risk of heart valve regurgitation after mediastinal radiation for Hodgkin's disease: an echocardiographic study. Heart 75:591–595
46. Heidenreich PA, Hancock SL, Lee BK (2003) Asymptomatic cardiac disease following mediastinal irradiation. J Am Coll Cardiol 42:743–749
47. Carlson RG, Mayfield W, Normann S (1991) Radiation-associated valvular disease. Chest 99:538–545
48. Hull MC, Morris CG, Pepine CJ (2003) Valvular dysfunction and carotid, subclavian, and coronary artery disease in survivors of hodgkin lymphoma treated with radiation therapy. JAMA 290:2831–2837
49. Gustavsson A, Bendahl PO, Cwikiel M (1999) No serious late cardiac effects after adjuvant radiotherapy following mastectomy in premenopausal women with early breast cancer. Int J Radiat Oncol Biol Phys 43:745–754
50. Orzan F, Brusca A, Gaita F (1993) Associated cardiac lesions in patients with radiation-induced complete heart block. Int J Cardiol 39:151–156
51. Slama MS, Le Guludec D, Sebag C (1991) Complete atrioventricular block following mediastinal irradiation: a report of six cases. PACE 14:1112–1118
52. Pohjola-Sintonen S, Totterman KJ, Kupari M (1990) Sick sinus syndrome as a complication of mediastinal radiation therapy. Cancer 65:2494–2496
53. Larsen RL, Jakacki RI, Vetter VL (1992) Electrocardiographic changes and arrhythmias after cancer therapy in children and young adults. Am J Cardiol 70:73–77
54. Hancock SL (1998) Cardiac toxicity after cancer therapy. Research issues in Cancer Survivorship Meeting, 3 Mar., National Cancer Institute, Bethesda, Maryland
55. Strender LE, Lindahl J, Larsson LE (1986) Incidence of heart disease and functional significance of changes in electrocardiogram 10 years after radiotherapy for breast cancer. Cancer 57:929–934
56. Carmel RJ, Kaplan HS (1976) Mantle irradiation in Hodgkin's disease. Cancer 37:2813–2815
57. Knobel H, Havard LJ, Brit LM (2001) Late medical complications and fatigue in Hodgkin's disease survivors. J Clin Oncol 19:3226–3233
58. Warda M, Khan A, Massumi A (1983) Radiation-induced valvular dysfunction. J Am Coll Cardiol 2:180–185
59. Van Renterghem D, Hamers J, De Shryver A (1985) Chylothorax after mantle irradiation for Hodgkin's disease. Respiration 48:188–189

60. Constine LS (1999) Late effects of cancer treatment. In: Halperin EC, Constine LS, Tarbell NJ, Kun LE (eds) Pediatric radiation oncology. Lippincott, Williams and Wilkins, New York, pp 457–537
61. Landier W, Bhatia S, Eshelman DA (2004) Development of risk-based guidelines for pediatric cancer survivors: the Children's Oncology Group Long-Term Follow-Up Guidelines from the Children's Oncology Group Late Effects Committee and Nursing Discipline. J Clin Oncol 22:4979–4990
62. Levitt GA, Jenney MEM (1998) The reproductive system after childhood cancer. Br J Obstet Gynaecol 105:946–953
63. Expert Panel on Detection Evaluation and Treatment of High Blood Cholesterol In Adults (2001) Executive summary of the third report of the National Cholesterol Education Program. JAMA 285:2486–2497
64. Bellenger NG, Burgess MI, Ray SG (2000) Comparison of left ventricular ejection fraction and volumes in heart failure by echocardiography, radionuclide ventriculography and cardiovascular magnetic resonance. Are they interchangeable? Eur Heart J 21:1387–1396
65. Pierga JY, Maunoury C, Valette H (1993) Follow-up thallium-201 scintigraphy after mantle field radiotherapy for Hodgkin's disease. Int J Radiat Oncol Biol Phys 25:871–876
66. Mancini DM, Eisen H, Kussmaul W (1991) Value of peak exercise oxygen consumption for the optimal timing of cardiac transplantation in ambulatory patients with heart failure. Circulation 83:778–786
67. Patel AR, Konstam MA (2001) Assessment of the patient with heart failure. In: Crawford MH, DiMarco JP (eds) Cardiology. Mosby, London, 5.2.1–10
68. Stevenson LW (1996) Selection and management of candidates for heart transplantation. [Review] [54 refs]. Curr Opin Cardiol 11:166–173, 1996
69. Handa N, McGregor CG, Danielson GK (1999) Coronary artery bypass grafting in patients with previous mediastinal radiation therapy. J Thorac Cardiovasc Surg 117:1136–1142
70. Handa N, McGregor CG, Danielson GK (2001) Valvular heart operation in patients with previous mediastinal radiation therapy. Ann Thorac Surg 71:1880–1884
71. Hicks GL Jr (1992) Coronary artery operation in radiation-associated atherosclerosis: long-term follow-up. Ann Thorac Surg 53:670–674
72. Gharagozloo F, Clements I, Mullany C (1992) Use of the internal mammary artery for myocardial revascularization in a patient with radiation-induced coronary artery disease. Mayo Clin Proc 67:1081–1084
73. van Son JA, Noyez L, van Asten W (1992) Use of internal mammary artery in myocardial revascularization after mediastinal irradiation. J Thorac Cardiovasc Surg 104:1539–1544
74. Reber D, Birnbaum DE, Tollenaere P (1995) Heart diseases following mediastinal irradiation: surgical management. Eur J of Cardiothorac Surg 9:202–205
75. Cotran RM, Kumar V, Robbins SL (1994) Robbins pathologic basis of disease, 5th ed. Harcourt Brace, London
76. Stewart JR, Fajardo LF, Gillette SM (1995) Radiation injury to the heart. Int J Radiat Oncol Biol Phys 31:1205–1211
77. Lipshultz SE, Sallan SE (1993) Cardiovascular abnormalities in long-term survivors of childhood malignancy. J Clin Oncol 11:1199–1203
78. Brosius FC, Waller BF, Roberts WC (1981) Radiation heart disease. Analysis of 16 young (aged 15–33 years) necropsy patients who received over 3,500 rads to the heart. Am J Med 70:519–530
79. Veinot JP, Edwards WD (1996) Pathology of radiation-induced heart disease: a surgical and autopsy study of 27 cases. Hum Pathol 27:766–773
80. Adams MJ, Constine LS, Lipshultz SE (2001) Radiation. In: Crawford MH, DiMarco JP (eds) Cardiology. Mosby, London, pp 8.15.1–8
81. Polikar R, Burger AG, Scherrer U (1993) The thyroid and the heart. Circulation 87:1435–1441
82. Glanzmann C, Kaufmann P, Jenni R (1998) Cardiac risk after mediastinal irradiation for Hodgkin's disease. Radiother Oncol 46:51–62
83. Lipshultz SE, Lipsitz SR, Mone SM (1995) Female sex and drug dose as risk factors for late cardiotoxic effects of doxorubicin therapy for childhood cancer. New Engl J Med 332:1738–1743
84. Perrault DJ, Levy M, Herman JD (1985) Echocardiographic abnormalities following cardiac radiation. J Clin Oncol 3:546–551
85. Cameron EH, Lipshultz SE, Tarbell NJ (1998) Cardiovascular disease in long-term survivors of pediatric Hodgkin's disease. Prog Pediatr Cardiol 8:139–144

Hypoxia-Mediated Chronic Normal Tissue Injury: A New Paradigm and Potential Strategies for Intervention

MITCHELL STEVEN ANSCHER and ZELJKO VUJASKOVIC

CONTENTS

8.1 Introduction 61
8.2 Hypoxia and Tissue Injury 61
8.3 The Hypoxia Paradigm of Chronic Radiation Injury 62
8.4 Potential Therapeutic Approaches 63
8.5 Conclusion 65
References 65

Summary

The tolerance of normal tissues to irradiation remains the major limitation to the use of ionizing radiation in the treatment of many malignancies. Recent progress in understanding the mechanisms underlying the development of late injury following cancer treatment points toward chronic hypoxia and oxidative stress as an important contributor to this problem. In this chapter, the authors review the evidence to support this new paradigm of late normal tissue injury and discuss potential approaches to the prevention and treatment of this condition.

8.1 Introduction

As the number of cancer survivors increases, the issue of long-term toxicity from treatment becomes increasingly important. The mechanisms responsible for sustaining the injured phenotype in normal tissues long after treatment has ended are currently under intense study. Recently, it has been demonstrated that the development and maintenance of chronic normal tissue hypoxia may be an important contributor to late normal tissue injury after radiation therapy. A new paradigm for late normal tissue injury, centered on chronic hypoxia, has been proposed (Fig. 8.1). This paradigm offers the opportunity for the development of new therapies directed against specific components of this injury pathway. Herein, we will discuss this new model, as well as possible avenues for intervention that arise from it.

M. S. ANSCHER, MD
Department of Radiation Oncology, Virginia Commonwealth University Medical Center, Box 980058, 401 College Street, Richmond, VA 23298-0058, USA
Z. VUJASKOVIC, MD, PhD
Department of Radiation Oncology, Duke University Medical Center, Box 3085 DUMC, Durham, NC 27710, USA

8.2 Hypoxia and Tissue Injury

Tissue hypoxia is a major regulatory signal for wound healing and tissue remodeling [16, 21]. Vascular damage from tissue injury often results in regions of low oxygen tension (hypoxia). Such hypoxic areas, which may be transient or chronic, are prevalent in malignant tumors [61], dermal wounds [2], atheromatous plaques [57], and in diabetic retinopathy [25]. Hypoxia also induces changes in membrane lipid composition, probably through the production of reactive oxygen species [12, 43]. These oxidants appear to arise from several processes, including superoxide leakage from mitochondrial respiration [10] and macrophage NADPH oxidase. Macrophages may also be attracted to hypoxic tissue and acti-

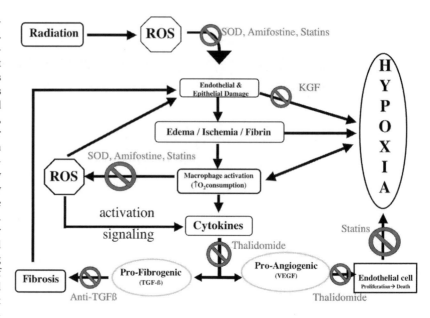

Fig. 8.1. Paradigm of hypoxia-mediated chronic lung injury. Initial tissue damage from radiation is generated by the direct action of reactive oxygen species (ROS) on DNA. This effect causes tissue injury including epithelial and endothelial cell damage, with an increase in vascular permeability, edema, and fibrin accumulation in the extracellular matrix. This tissue injury is followed by an inflammatory response including macrophage accumulation and activation. Macrophages, along with other inflammatory cells, are attracted to an area of injury or evolving inflammation. The majority of macrophages in lung are derived from circulating monocytes that enter the lung in response to inflammation. These macrophages are able to release a number of cytokines and ROS. Both vascular changes as well as an increase in oxygen consumption (due to macrophage activation) contribute to the development of hypoxia. Hypoxia further stimulates production of ROS, and profibrogenic and proangiogenic cytokines. This response to hypoxia perpetuates tissue damage leading to fibrosis via TGFß production and stimulates angiogenesis through VEGF production. While attempting to respond to the proliferative stimulus of VEGF, endothelial cells die as a result of previously accumulated radiation damage. Thus, hypoxia continuously perpetuates a non-healing tissue response leading to chronic radiation injury. This injury pathway offers numerous potential targets for therapeutic intervention

vated by products of hypoxic tissue injury [19, 27, 50]. In addition, hypoxia stimulates the release of proinflammatory, profibrotic, and proangiogenic cytokines by a variety of cells involved in tissue repair [40, 45, 53], leading to increased vascular permeability, leukocyte migration, collagen deposition, and angiogenesis [26, 56, 67]. Hypoxia also upregulates several transcription factors, including p53, and triggers p53-dependent apoptosis [24, 59].

8.3
The Hypoxia Paradigm of Chronic Radiation Injury

The biological effects of ionizing radiation begin with the radiolysis of water leading to the generation of reactive oxygen species (ROS), such as superoxide (O_2-), hydrogen peroxide (H_2O_2), and the hydroxyl radical (OH–) [51]. These ROS damage tissue directly through interaction with DNA, as well as via cytokine induction and activation [3, 14, 52, 54]. The targets of ROS-mediated injury include the endothelial cell, resulting in increased permeability, edema, and fibrin accumulation in the extracellular matrix [34]. Tissue injury leads to an inflammatory response including accumulation and activation of macrophages [58]. The majority of macrophages appear to be derived from circulating monocytes that enter the injured tissue in response to inflammatory signaling [28]. These macrophages in turn release a number of cytokines and ROS [17, 49]. The presence of activated macrophages also leads to increased oxygen consumption in the tissues. Thus, a state of decreased oxygen delivery, due to vascular damage, and increased oxygen consumption, by activated macrophages, develops in the injured tissue leading to hypoxia [34, 62] (Fig. 8.2). This hypoxic state further stimulates production of ROS (Fig. 8.3), proinflammatory, profibrotic, and proangiogenic cytokines [22, 23, 31, 32, 56], which perpetuates tissue damage leading to fibrosis via transforming growth factor ß (TGFβ) production [8]. In an attempt to respond to the proliferative stimulus from vascular endothelial growth factor (VEGF), endothelial cells damaged from prior radiation-induced injury die, further decreasing perfusion to the injured tissue. Thus, hypoxia continuously perpetuates a non-healing response leading to chronic radiation injury.

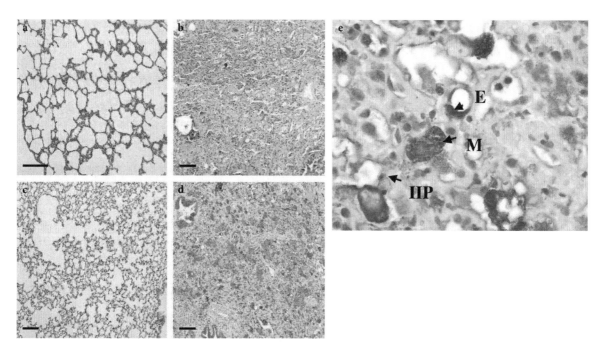

Fig. 8.2a–e. Evidence for the presence of hypoxic regions in normal lung following a single dose of 28 Gy to the right hemithorax in Fisher rats. Masson trichrome stain demonstrates very little fibrous tissue development at 6 weeks after irradiation (**a**), but widespread fibrosis is evident in irradiated lung by 6 months (**b**). Similarly, intravenous injection of the hypoxia marker pimonidazole indicates little hypoxia at 6 weeks after irradiation (**c**), but widespread hypoxia is evident in irradiated lung at 6 months (**d**). A higher power view (**e**) demonstrates that hypoxia is evident primarily in endothelial cells (*E*) and macrophages (*M*). *IIP*, type-II pneumocyte. Each black bar is 100 μm

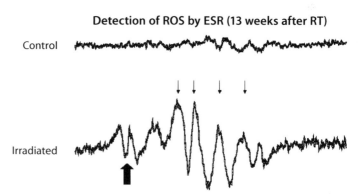

Fig. 8.3. Demonstration of the presence of reactive oxygen species (ROS) in irradiated lung tissue using the technique of electron spin resonance (ESR) 13 weeks after single-dose irradiation. The *thick black arrow* indicates the presence of ROS. The peaks denoted by the *thin arrows* represent artifact

8.4
Potential Therapeutic Approaches

The hypoxia paradigm of chronic radiation injury diagrammed in Figure 8.1 offers several potential targets for intervention. As noted above, sustained overproduction of ROS appears to be one important component of late normal tissue injury. One of the more promising approaches to reducing the impact of this oxidative stress resulting from radiation exposure is through the superoxide dismutase (SOD) pathway. The SODs are a family of metalloprotein enzymes that play an important role in protection from oxidative damage. They function by catalyzing the conversion of superoxide to hydrogen peroxide and oxygen [51]. Hydrogen peroxide is further reduced by catalase and/or glutathione peroxidase to water and oxygen [47, 60]. It exists naturally in three forms: mitochondrial, cytoplasmic, and extracellular. Several different approaches have been used to test the efficacy of SOD as a radioprotector. Kang et al. have demonstrated, using a mouse model engineered to constitutively overexpress extracellular SOD, a significant reduction in the expression of the profibrogenic cytokine TGFß with a corresponding decrease in pulmonary fibrosis [29]. The transgenic animals also had a significantly lower breathing frequency compared with irradiated controls. Using exogenously administered SOD, either in the form of gene therapy [18] or an SOD mimetic compound [63], others have also demonstrated significant pulmonary radioprotection in experimental animal models. In humans, SOD has been shown to reverse late soft tissue fibrosis in a prospective randomized trial [13]. While SOD has not been tried in humans for the treatment or prevention of radiation-induced lung injury, this approach seems promising. The other major free radical scavenger, which has been tested in humans, is amifostine. Several small randomized trials have demonstrated significant pulmonary radioprotection for this drug [33]. More recently, a larger randomized study from the Radiation Therapy Oncology Group (RTOG) failed to find a protective effect in the lung for amifostine [64]. The design of this RTOG study has been criticized in that the radiation was given twice per day, and yet amifostine, which has a short half-life, was only given once per day. Thus, despite the presence of convincing animal data, the question of the efficacy of amifostine as a pulmonary radioprotector remains unresolved.

Since numerous cytokines are important in the inflammatory and fibrotic response that develops after radiation exposure, targeting one or more of these cytokines is a logical approach to the prevention and treatment of radiation injury. Possible strategies could include the use of agents that are specifically targeted against a single cytokine, or agents that are non-specific and may exert an effect via interfering with the actions of multiple cytokines involved in the injury process. The profibrotic cytokine TGFß has been shown to be critical to the production of excess connective tissue in a number of fibrosing conditions, including after exposure to radiation [1, 9, 11]. TGFß is secreted in a biologically inactive form and, once activated [36, 41], TGFß binds to its type-II transmembrane receptor as the first step in the initiation of its signaling pathway [37]. In animal models of radiation injury, soluble forms of this type-II receptor have been administered via a gene therapy approach and have been shown to be effective in reducing both radiation-induced intestinal and pulmonary injury [44, 48, 66]. Similarly, blocking the TGFß signaling pathway, in this case by using mice that are deficient in the Smad 3 component of the pathway, has also been shown to protect against radiation-induced soft tissue fibrosis [20]. Thus, anti-TGFß therapy appears to be a promising approach to the prevention of radiation-induced injury. Whether this cytokine can be targeted to reverse established injury remains to be determined.

A second strategy for targeting cytokines to prevent radiation-induced normal tissue injury is through the use of agents that non-specifically inhibit the actions of more than one cytokine. Many drugs have an effect on cytokine pathways, and, since these pathways are involved in multiple pathologic processes, some of these agents are being investigated as potential radioprotectors. Among the commercially available drugs currently under investigation in the clinic are thalidomide and the 3-hydroxy-3-methylglutaryl coenzyme A (HMG-CoA) reductase inhibitors (statins). Thalidomide and its analogs, the selective cytokine inhibitory drugs, affect the production of several cytokines involved in the development of normal tissue injury after radiation therapy, including tumor necrosis factor α (TNFα), vascular endothelial growth factor (VEGF), basic fibroblast growth factor (bFGF), and several of the interleukins (IL), but it is likely that the effect of thalidomide on these cytokines varies depending on the clinical circumstances in which it is used (reviewed in [38]). The drug has been shown to be active against advanced non-small-cell lung cancer (NSCLC) [39]. Although no preclinical data exist demonstrating normal tissue radioprotection, given its efficacy against this disease and its broad anticytokine activity profile, thalidomide is currently undergoing phase I testing to assess its ability to modulate radiation-induced lung injury.

The statins are among the most widely prescribed drugs in the US. In addition to their lipid lowering properties, these agents promote vascular thromboresistance [55] and affect immunity, inflammation, intracellular signaling pathways, and oxidative stress, which influences cell migration and proliferation independent of effects on plasma lipids [6, 7, 30, 42, 46]. Because of their vascular protective properties, statins are currently in clinical trials in Europe to assess whether they can reduce the incidence of large vessel injury and stroke following head and neck irradiation. These agents have also been recently demonstrated to protect against the development of late radiation-induced lung injury in a murine model [65], probably through a mechanism that involves reduction in recruitment of macrophages and lymphocytes to the site of injury. A clinical trial of simvastatin as a pulmonary radioprotectant is under development through the International Atomic Energy Agency. Thus, statins may prove to be useful in protecting against radiation injury in numerous tissues. Whether they can reverse established injury is not known.

Finally, most approaches to radiation protection have focused on events taking place in the stromal compartment. This philosophy has evolved, in part, because until recently there was little that could be done to protect irradiated epithelium. With the development of recombinant growth factors, it is now possible to pharmacologically stimulate epithelial proliferation; this approach has been shown to be effective in the treatment of acute mucosal reactions resulting from irradiation for head and neck cancer [15]. Recently, recombinant human keratinocyte growth factor (rhuKGF) has been shown to protect against late radiation-induced pulmonary injury in an animal model, in part via downregulation of the TGFß-mediated fibrosis pathway [35]. These results suggest that epithelial-stromal signaling interactions may play an important role in the development and prevention of late radiation-induced normal tissue injury [4, 5]. KGF has not yet been tested in humans to determine whether it can prevent late radiation injury.

8.5 Conclusion

In summary, chronic oxidative stress leading to normal tissue hypoxia appears to be an important factor in the development of chronic injury after exposure to radiation therapy. Multiple targets along this injury pathway may be susceptible to disruption, with a consequential reduction in the severity of injury. New agents are under development, and commercially available drugs are currently entering clinical trials to determine their efficacy in preventing radiation injury. More work is needed to develop drugs that can reverse established late damage. Thus, in the near future, clinicians should have more options for treating long-term side effects in the ever-expanding population of cancer survivors.

References

1. Anscher MS, Crocker IR, Jirtle RL (1990) Transforming growth factor-beta 1 expression in irradiated liver. Radiat Res 122:77–85
2. Arnold F, West D, Kumar S (1987) Wound healing: the effect of macrophage and tumour derived angiogenesis factors on skin graft vascularization. Br J Exp Pathol 68:569–574
3. Barcellos-Hoff M, Dix T (1996) Redox-mediated activation of latent transforming growth factor-ß1. Mol Endocrinol 10:1077–1083
4. Barcellos-Hoff M (1998) How do tissues respond to damage at the cellular level? The role of cytokines in irradiated tissues. Radiat Res 150:S109–S120
5. Barcellos-Hoff MH, Brooks AL (2001) Extracellular signaling through the microenvironment: a hypothesis relating carcinogenesis, bystander effects, and genomic instability. Radiat Res 156:618–627
6. Bellosta S, Bernini F, Ferri N et al (1998) Direct vascular effects of HMG-CoA reductase inhibitors. Atherosclerosis 137[Suppl]:101–109
7. Bellosta S, Via D, Canavesi M et al (1998) HMG-CoA reductase inhibitors reduce MMP-9 secretion by macrophages. Arterioscler Thromb Vasc Biol 18:1671–1678
8. Benson J, Poulsen H, Hougaard S et al (1998) TGFß and cancer in other organs. Lung cancer. In: Benson J (ed) TGFß and cancer. RG Landes Company, London, pp 155–158
9. Broekelmann TJ, Limper AH, Colby TV et al (1991) Transforming growth factor beta-1 is present at sites of extracellular matrix gene expression in human pulmonary fibrosis. Proc Natl Acad Sci USA 88:6642–6646
10. Cadenas E, Boveris A, Ragan CI et al (1977) Production of superoxide radicals and hydrogen peroxide by NADH-ubiquinone reductase and ubiquinol-cytochrome c reductase from beef-heart mitochondria. Arch Biochem Biophys 180:248–257
11. Castilla A, Prieto J, Fausto N (1991) Transforming growth factors beta-1 and alpha in chronic liver disease – effects of interferon alpha therapy. N Eng J Med 324:993–940
12. Coleman SE, Duggan J, Hackett RL (1976) Plasma membrane changes in freeze-fractured rat kidney cortex following renal ischemia. Lab Invest 35:63–70
13. Delanian S, Baillet F, Huart J et al (1994) Successful treatment of radiation-induced fibrosis using liposomal Cu/Zn superoxide dismutase: clinical trial. Radiother Oncol 32:12–20
14. Dent P, Yacoub A, Contessa J et al (2003) Stress and radiation-induced activation of multiple intracellular signaling pathways. Radiat Res 159:283–300
15. Dorr W, Spekl K, Farrell CL (2002) Amelioration of acute oral mucositis by keratinocyte growth factor: fractionated irradiation. Int J Radiat Oncol Biol Phys 54:245–251
16. Dvorak HF (1986) Tumors: wounds that do not heal. Similarities between tumor stroma generation and wound healing. N Engl J Med 315:1650–1659
17. Elias JA, Gustilo K, Freundlich B (1988) Human alveolar macrophage and blood monocyte inhibition of fibroblast proliferation. Evidence for synergy between interleukin-1 and tumor necrosis factor. Am Rev Respir Dis 138:1595–1603
18. Epperly MW, Defilippi S, Sikora C et al (2000) Intratracheal injection of manganese superoxide dismutase (Mn-

SOD) plasmid/liposomes protects normal lung but not orthotopic tumors from irradiation. Gene Ther 7:1011–1018
19. Esser P, Heimann K, Wiedemann P (1993) Macrophages in proliferative vitreoretinopathy and proliferative diabetic retinopathy: differentiation of subpopulations. Br J Ophthalmol 77:731–733
20. Flanders KC, Sullivan CD, Fujii M et al (2002) Mice lacking Smad3 are protected against cutaneous injury induced by ionizing radiation. Am J Pathol 160:1057–1068
21. Folkman J (1995) Angiogenesis in cancer, vascular, rheumatoid and other disease. Nat Med 1:27–31
22. Frater-Schroder M, Muller G, Birchmeier W et al (1986) Transforming growth factor-beta inhibits endothelial cell proliferation. Biochem Biophys Res Commun 137:295–302
23. Frater-Schroder M, Risau W, Hallmann R et al (1987) Tumor necrosis factor type alpha, a potent inhibitor of endothelial cell growth in vitro, is angiogenic in vivo. Proc Natl Acad Sci USA 84:5277–5281
24. Graeber TG, Osmanian C, Jacks T et al (1996) Hypoxia-mediated selection of cells with diminished apoptotic potential in solid tumours. Nature 379:88–91
25. Hammes HP, Lin J, Bretzel RG et al (1998) Upregulation of the vascular endothelial growth factor/vascular endothelial growth factor receptor system in experimental background diabetic retinopathy of the rat. Diabetes 47:401–406
26. Haroon ZA, Raleigh JA, Greenberg CS et al (2000) Early wound healing exhibits cytokine surge without evidence of hypoxia. Ann Surg 231:137–147
27. Hunt TK, Knighton DR, Thakral KK et al (1984) Studies on inflammation and wound healing: angiogenesis and collagen synthesis stimulated in vivo by resident and activated wound macrophages. Surgery 96:48–54
28. Johnston CJ, Williams JP, Okunieff P et al (2002) Radiation-induced pulmonary fibrosis: examination of chemokine and chemokine receptor families. Radiat Res 157:256–265
29. Kang S, Rabbani Z, Folz R et al (2002) Overexpression of extracellular superoxide dismutase protects mice from radiation induced lung injury. Int J Radiat Oncol Biol Phys 54:78
30. Kinlay S, Selwyn AP, Delagrange D et al (1996) Biological mechanisms for the clinical success of lipid-lowering in coronary artery disease and the use of surrogate endpoints. Curr Opin Lipidol 7:389–397
31. Knighton DR, Hunt TK, Scheuenstuhl H et al (1983) Oxygen tension regulates the expression of angiogenesis factor by macrophages. Science 221:1283–1285
32. Koch AE, Polverini PJ, Kunkel SL et al (1992) Interleukin-8 as a macrophage-derived mediator of angiogenesis. Science 258:1798–1801
33. Komaki R, Lee JS, Milas L et al (2004) Effects of amifostine on acute toxicity from concurrent chemotherapy and radiotherapy for inoperable non-small-cell lung cancer: report of a randomized comparative trial. Int J Radiat Oncol Biol Phys 58:1369–1377
34. Li Y-Q, Ballinger J, Nordal R et al (2001) Hypoxia in radiation-induced blood-spinal cord barrier breakdown. Cancer Res 61:3348–3354
35. Liguang C, Larrier N, Rabbani ZN et al (2003) Assessment of the protective effect of keratinocyte growth factor on radiation-induced pulmonary toxicity in rats. Int J Radiat Oncol Biol Phys 57:S162
36. Lyons RM, Gentry LE, Purchio AF et al (1990) Mechanism of activation of latent recombinant transforming growth factor ß1 by plasmin. J Cell Biol 110:1361–1367
37. Massague J (1998) TGF-beta signal transduction. Annu Rev Biochem 67:753–791
38. Matthews SJ, McCoy C (2003) Thalidomide: a review of approved and investigational uses. Clin Ther 25:342–395
39. Merchant J, Kim K, Mehta M et al (2000) Pilot and safety trial of Carboplatin, Paclitaxel, and Thalidomide in advanced non-small cell lung cancer. Clin Lung Cancer 2:48–52
40. Minchenko A, Bauer T, Salceda S et al (1994) Hypoxic stimulation of vascular endothelial growth factor expression in vitro and in vivo. Lab Invest 71:374–379
41. Munger J, Huang X, Kawakatsu H et al (1999) The integrin vß6 binds and activates latent TGFß1: a mechanism for regulating pulmonary inflammation and fibrosis. Cell 96:319–328
42. Nakagami H, Jensen KS, Liao JK (2003) A novel pleiotropic effect of statins: prevention of cardiac hypertrophy by cholesterol-independent mechanisms. Ann Med 35:398–403
43. Nakanishi K, Tajima F, Nakamura A et al (1995) Effects of hypobaric hypoxia on antioxidant enzymes in rats. J Physiol 489:869–876
44. Nishioka A, Ogawa Y, Mima T et al (2004) Histopathologic amelioration of fibroproliferative change in rat irradiated lung using soluble transforming growth factor-beta (TGF-beta) receptor mediated by adenoviral vector. Int J Radiat Oncol Biol Phys 58:1235–1241
45. Patel B, Khaliq A, Jarvis-Evans J et al (1994) Oxygen regulation of TGF-beta 1 mRNA in human hepatoma (Hep G2) cells. Biochem Mol Biol Int 34:639–644
46. Perez-Guerrero C, Alvarez de Sotomayor M, Jimenez L et al (2003) Effects of simvastatin on endothelial function after chronic inhibition of nitric oxide synthase by L-NAME. J Cardiovasc Pharmacol 42:204–210
47. Quinlan T, Spivack S, Mossman BT (1994) Regulation of antioxidant enzymes in lung after oxidant injury. Environ Health Perspect 102[Suppl]2:79–87
48. Rabbani ZN, Anscher MS, Zhang X et al (2003) Soluble TGFß type II receptor gene therapy ameliorates acute radiation-induced pulmonary injury in rats. Int J Radiat Biol Oncol Phys 57:563–572
49. Rappolee DA, Mark D, Banda MJ et al (1988) Wound macrophages express TGF-alpha and other growth factors in vivo: analysis by mRNA phenotyping. Science 241:708–712
50. Remensnyder JP, Majno G (1968) Oxygen gradients in healing wounds. Am J Pathol 52:301–323
51. Riley PA: Free radicals in biology: oxidative stress and the effects of ionizing radiation. Int J Radiat Biol 65:27–33, 1994
52. Rubin P, Johnston CJ, Williams JP et al (1995) A perpetual cascade of cytokines post irradiation leads to pulmonary fibrosis. Int J Radiat Oncol Biol Phys 33:99–109
53. Scannell G, Waxman K, Kaml GJ et al (1993) Hypoxia induces a human macrophage cell line to release tumor necrosis factor-alpha and its soluble receptors in vitro. J Surg Res 54:281–285

54. Schieffer B, Luchtefeld M, Braun S et al (2000) Role of NAD(P)H oxidase in angiotensin II-induced JAK/STAT signaling and cytokine induction. Circ Res 87:1195–1201
55. Shi J, Wang J, Zheng H et al (2003) Statins increase thrombomodulin expression and function in human endothelial cells by a nitric oxide-dependent mechanism and counteract tumor necrosis factor alpha-induced thrombomodulin downregulation. Blood Coagul Fibrinolysis 14:575–585
56. Shweiki D, Itin A, Soffer D et al (1992) Vascular endothelial growth factor induced by hypoxia may mediate hypoxia-initiated angiogenesis. Nature 359:843–845
57. Simanonok JP (1996) Non-ischemic hypoxia of the arterial wall is a primary cause of atherosclerosis. Med Hypotheses 46:155–161
58. Stone HB, Coleman CN, Anscher MS et al (2003) Effects of radiation on normal tissue: consequences and mechanisms. Lancet Oncol 4:529–536
59. Sun Y, Oberley LW (1996) Redox regulation of transcriptional activators. Free Radic Biol Med 21:335–348
60. Tsan MF (1997) Superoxide dismutase and pulmonary oxygen toxicity. Proc Soc Exp Biol Med 214:107–113
61. Vaupel P, Schlenger K, Knoop C et al (1991) Oxygenation of human tumors: evaluation of tissue oxygen distribution in breast cancers by computerized O2 tension measurements. Cancer Res 51:3316–3322
62. Vujaskovic Z, Anscher M, Feng Q-F et al (2001) Radiation-induced hypoxia may perpetuate late normal tissue injury. Int J Radiat Oncol Biol Phys 50:851–855
63. Vujaskovic Z, Batinic-Haberle I, Rabbani Z et al (2002) A small molecular weight catalytic metalloporphyrin antioxidant with superoxide dismutase (SOD) mimetic properties protects lungs from radiation-induced injury. Free Radic Biol Med 33:857
64. Werner-Wasik M, Scott C, Movsas B et al (2003) Amifostine as a mucosal protectant in patients with locally advanced non-small cell lung cancer (NSCLC) receiving intensive chemotherapy and thoracic radiotherapy (RT): results of the Radiation Therapy Oncology Group (RTOG) 90–01 study. Int J Radiat Oncol Biol Phys 57:S216
65. Williams JP, Hernady E, Johnston CJ et al (2004) Effect of administration of lovastatin on the development of late pulmonary effects after whole-lung irradiation in a murine model. Radiat Res 161:560–567
66. Zheng H, Wang J, Koteliansky V, et al (2000) Recombinant soluble transforming growth factor ß type II receptor ameliorates radiation enteropathy in mice. Gastroenterology 119:1286–1296
67. Zhong Z, Arteel GE, Connor HD et al (1998) Cyclosporin A increases hypoxia and free radical production in rat kidneys: prevention by dietary glycine. Am J Physiol 275:595–604

Prevention and Treatment of Radiation Injuries – The Role of the Renin-Angiotensin System

Eric P. Cohen, Melissa M. Joines, and John E. Moulder

CONTENTS

9.1 Introduction 69
9.2 The Renin-Angiotensin System 69
9.3 The Case of Radiation Nephropathy 71
9.4 Non-renal Tissues 73
9.5 Clinical Implications 73
9.6 Conclusions 74
References 75

9.1 Introduction

Inexorable progression is the traditional view of late normal tissue radiation injury [1]. Symptomatic treatments may be used, but, until recently, effective treatment or mitigation of normal tissue radiation injury was not possible. Recent studies in multiple models show that this is no longer the case [2–4]. The involvement of the renin-angiotensin system (RAS) in the normal tissue response to irradiation is of particular interest, because antagonists of the RAS are effective in mitigation and treatment of many normal tissue radiation injuries (Table 9.1).

Summary

The renin-angiotensin system, local or systemic, plays a key role in normal tissue radiation injury. Angiotensin converting enzyme (ACE) inhibitors, which act to attenuate the conversion of angiotensin I to angiotensin II, are beneficial in mitigating experimental renal, lung, or brain normal tissue radiation injury. The benefit of ACE inhibitors and angiotensin II blockers has been particularly well documented in experimental radiation nephropathy, for either mitigation or treatment. The mechanism for this benefit remains incompletely understood. In particular, control of hypertension, proteinuria, or radiation-induced cell proliferation alone does not appear to determine the benefit of ACE inhibitors or angiotensin II blockers. Nonetheless, the significant experimental benefit of those agents fully justifies their use in human radiation nephropathy. Clinical trials using ACE inhibitors are underway in subjects undergoing radiation-based bone marrow transplantation and also in subjects undergoing curative radiotherapy for lung cancer.

E. P. Cohen, MD
Department of Medicine, Nephrology Division, Medical College of Wisconsin, 9200 W. Wisconsin Ave., Milwaukee, WI 53226, USA

M. M. Joines, BS
Department of Medicine and Radiation Oncology, Medical College of Wisconsin, 9200 W. Wisconsin Ave., Milwaukee, WI 53226, USA

J. E. Moulder, PhD
Professor of Radiation Oncology, Director, Center for Medical Countermeasures Against Radiologicol Terrorism, Medical College of Wisconsin, 8701 Watertown Plank Road, Milwaukee, WI 53226, USA

9.2 The Renin-Angiotensin System

RAS was long understood as an endocrine pathway that had a central role in the physiology of the kidneys and blood circulation (Fig. 9.1). In a classical negative feedback loop, a fall in arterial blood pressure leads to renin release by the kidneys, and renin cleaves angiotensinogen to angiotensin I, which is then converted by angiotensin converting enzyme

Table 9.1. Suppression of the RAS and radiation injuries

Reference	Drug	Schedule, endpoint, and system
[31]	Captopril (ACE inhibitor)	Mitigation of acute renal injury (pig)
[32]	Captopril	Mitigation of pulmonary dysfunction (rat)
[33]	Other ACE inhibitors	Mitigation of pulmonary dysfunction (rat)
[34]	Captopril	Mitigation of acute and late skin damage (rat)
[35]	Captopril	Treatment of chronic renal injury (rat)
[10]	Captopril	Mitigation of chronic renal injury (rat)
[11]	Other ACE inhibitors	Mitigation of chronic renal injury (rat)
[36]	ACE inhibitors	Treatment of renal injury after BMT (human)
[18]	L-158809 (AT_1 blocker)	Mitigation and treatment of chronic renal injury (rat)
[37]	L-158809 (AT_1 blocker)	Mitigation of chronic lung injury (rat)
[16]	High dietary salt	Mitigation of chronic renal injury (rat)
[27]	Losartan (AT_1 blocker)	Treatment of chronic renal injury (human)
[38]	PD-123319 (AT_2 blocker)	Mitigation of chronic renal injury (rat)
[23]	Ramipril (ACE inhibitor)	Mitigation of optic neuropathy (rat)

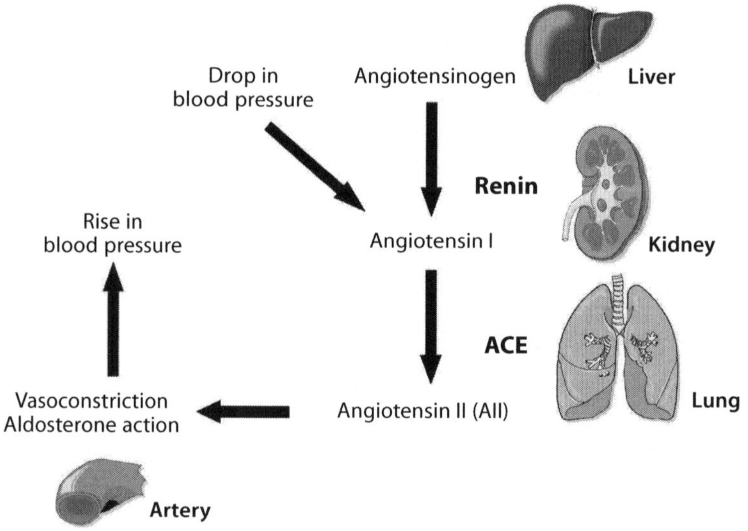

Fig. 9.1. A simplified version of the endocrine renin-angiotensin system (RAS). The conversion of angiotensinogen by renin is shown as mediated by a fall in blood pressure. The resulting production of angiotensin I (A_I) leads to production of angiotensin II (A_{II}), via angiotensin converting enzyme (ACE), and A_{II} acts to increase the blood pressure, thus turning off the initial stimulus

(ACE) to angiotensin II (A_{II}), an octapeptide vasoconstrictor. This raises the blood pressure, which turns off the stimulus to renin release. A_{II} also stimulates aldosterone secretion by the adrenal glands, and that mineralocorticoid acts on kidneys to promote salt retention, which in turn assists in raising the blood pressure.

This simple system is in reality much more complex (Fig. 9.2). There are non-ACE pathways for angiotensin synthesis, there are at least two types of A_{II} receptor, and some tissues have entire RAS within them (so-called paracrine systems). All the components of the RAS, from renin to A_{II} receptors, for instance, are present in heart and kidneys [5].

As the RAS has become better known, pharmaceuticals have been developed that act on it. One of the earliest, teprotide, was isolated from snake venom almost 40 years ago [6]. From this was derived the drug captopril, which inhibits ACE, thereby antagonizing the RAS. Captopril and its congeners, such as

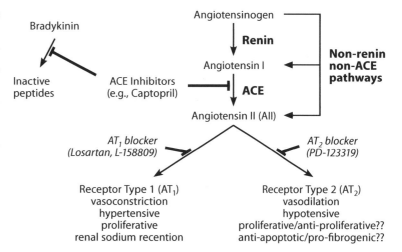

Fig. 9.2. A more detailed diagram of the RAS. The addition of conversion pathways other than renin and ACE are shown, as is part of the bradykinin pathway. The presence of two types of A_{II} receptors is also shown, along with their antagonists. It is likely that there are additional types of A_{II} receptor. The paracrine (tissue-localized) RAS adds additional complexity, which is not shown

enalapril and lisinopril, are in common clinical use today for treatment of hypertension, renal disease, and heart failure. It is likely that their benefits depend on both the control of blood pressure and on antagonism of the RAS (endocrine and paracrine).

In the case of diabetic renal disease, so-called diabetic nephropathy, captopril and other ACE inhibitors were shown to be effective in treatment of patients with established renal disease in the early 1990s [7]. More recently, the focus has shifted towards earlier intervention, before loss of kidney function. There are similar distinctions in the approach to radiation injuries (Fig. 9.3).

Use of ACE inhibitors and A_{II} blockers in treatment and mitigation of normal tissue radiation injuries are summarized on Table 9.1. Clearly, these agents are effective in more than one tissue and in more than one animal species. That effect is, however, not totally generalizable, because ACE inhibitors are not effective in mitigating gastrointestinal [8] or bone marrow injury in rats [9]. Nonetheless, the weight of the data have overturned the traditional view that normal tissue radiation injuries are untreatable.

9.3
The Case of Radiation Nephropathy

We have investigated the mechanism of action whereby ACE inhibitors and A_{II}-blockers mitigate and treat radiation nephropathy. These might include the antihypertensive action of these drugs,

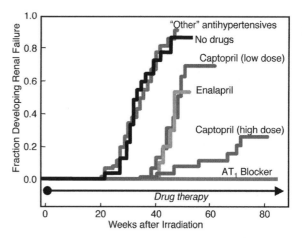

Fig. 9.3. Effect of antihypertensive therapies on the development of experimental radiation nephropathy. Actuarial incidence curves of the development of renal failure are shown for rats that received 17 Gy (in six fractions) plus BMT and were treated with: high and low dose captopril, enalapril, an A_{II} type-1 receptor antagonist (L-158,809), or various other antihypertensives that act by mechanisms not directly related to A_{II} activity

their effect on urinary protein, their effect on renal cell proliferation, or their blockade of radiation-activated RAS.

We use a total-body irradiation (TBI) model to establish radiation nephropathy. Barrier-maintained rats undergo 17 Gy TBI in six equal fractions over 3 days, followed by bone marrow transplantation (BMT) from a syngeneic litter mate [10]. Renal failure is the major normal tissue toxicity in this model. It is marked by proteinuria, hypertension, and azotemia. We have used multiple antihypertensive agents in attempts to mitigate and treat radiation nephropathy in this model. Anti-hypertensive drugs that do not act on the RAS are ineffective at slowing the progression to renal failure, as shown in Figure 9.3. On the other hand, captopril and its non-thiol congener, enalapril, significantly slow progression in this model [11]. It is worth noting that the beneficial effect of low-dose captopril occurs without blunting the proteinuria in this model. Thus, the benefits of ACE inhibitors in radiation nephropathy appear to occur independently of controlling proteinuria, and antihypertensives that do not interact with the RAS do not protect against radiation nephropathy. What is also noteworthy is that the benefits of captopril in this model occur at a dose which is compatible with human doses used in the clinic, when factored per body surface area.

In addition, captopril does not have to be present at the time of irradiation to exert a long-term beneficial effect in experimental radiation nephropathy. We showed that one could delay the start of captopril therapy until 25 days after TBI and still achieve excellent long-term benefits, i.e., mitigation of radiation nephropathy [12]. These data show that captopril is not acting as a classical radioprotector.

Because A_{II} is a growth promoter for kidney cells [13] we tested the hypothesis that the beneficial effects of ACE inhibitors or A_{II} blockers was dependent on their anti-proliferative action. Renal epithelial cell proliferation is well documented in radiation nephropathy and could play a mechanistic role [14]. Using our 17-Gy TBI-BMT model, we tested this hypothesis by quantifying renal cellular proliferation using immunohistochemistry for proliferating cell nuclear antigen (PCNA). Continuous use of the A_{II} blocker, L-158,809, from the time of irradiation onward, significantly reduced tubular epithelial proliferation to below that of rats receiving only radiation (Fig. 9.4) [15]. However, subsequent studies using the same model do not support the tubular cell proliferation hypothesis. In these studies, we showed that a high-salt diet, appropriately timed, had a long-term beneficial effect in radiation nephropathy and that this coincided with suppression of the RAS [16]. We then tested whether a high-salt diet exerted this beneficial effect via a reduction in renal tubular cell proliferation; it did not (JE Moulder and EP Cohen, unpublished observation).

The involvement of the RAS in radiation nephropathy has been further tested by analysis of its components. Serum renin does not change during

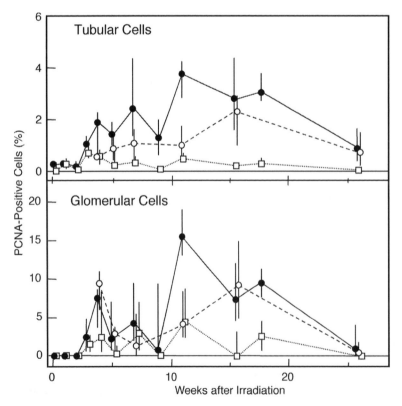

Fig. 9.4. Time course of proliferation rates, as assessed by PCNA labeling, of renal tubular and glomerular cells in rats given 17 Gy (in six fractions) alone (*solid circles*) or 17 Gy (in six fractions) plus an A_{II} type-1 receptor antagonist, L-158,809 (*open circles*), compared with unirradiated controls (*open squares*). The data are shown as medians with 20%–80% ranges. (Reproduced from [15] with permission)

the first 6 weeks after irradiation and is below normal at 17 weeks after 17 Gy TBI [17]. During the 3- to 9-week interval after TBI, when ACE inhibitors and A_{II} blockers are most effective [18, 19], neither whole blood A_{II} nor intrarenal A_{II} levels are different from those of age-matched, unirradiated rats [17]. During that same interval, there appears to be no change in saturable renal A_{II} receptor binding (Fig. 9.5). Thus, the beneficial effect of ACE inhibitors and A_{II} blockers in radiation nephropathy appears to occur in the setting of a normally active RAS.

It has been proposed that the benefit of blockade of the angiotensin type-I (AT_1) receptor derives from the unopposed action of A_{II} on the angiotensin type-2 (AT_2) receptor [20]. We tested this and found the opposite effect – addition of the AT_2 antagonist enhanced the beneficial effect of AT_1 blockade (Fig. 9.6). Studies of AT_2 and AT_1 receptors have not shown their upregulation in irradiated kidney (JE Moulder and EP Cohen, unpublished observation).

9.4
Non-renal Tissues

Attenuation of radiation pneumopathy by captopril and other ACE inhibitors was shown by Ward et al. [21, 22] over 10 years ago. These were studies in which drug was started prior to the time of irradiation and continued indefinitely. Therapy studies of radiation pneumopathy, using drug starting when there is established injury, have not been done.

A recent study by Kim et al. [23] showed significant attenuation of radiation-induced optic neuropathy, as measured anatomically and by visual evoked potentials (Fig. 9.7). Again, this is a mitigation, not a treatment study.

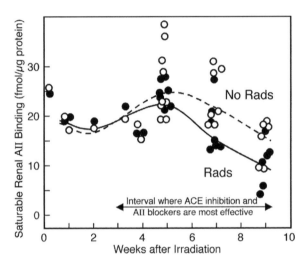

Fig. 9.5. Time course of A_{II} binding in kidney microsomes obtained from irradiated (17 Gy in six fractions) and control rats. Microsomes obtained from irradiated rats (*solid circles*) did not have different A_{II} binding compared to that of unirradiated control rats (*open circles*), specifically during the interval in which ACE inhibitors and A_{II} type-1 antagonists are effective in attenuating long-term injury

9.5
Clinical Implications

We have linked chronic renal failure after BMT to the TBI that is often given as part of the pre-

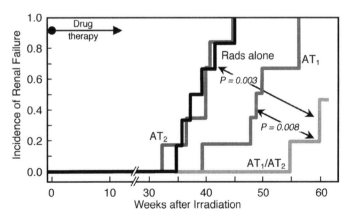

Fig. 9.6. Effect of A_{II} antagonists on the development of experimental radiation nephropathy. Actuarial incidence curves of the development of renal failure are shown. The type-1 or the type-2 A_{II} (PD123319) antagonists were used until 12 weeks after 17 Gy irradiation plus BMT. The A_{II} type-1 antagonist significantly delayed the development of renal failure. By itself, the A_{II} type-2 antagonist had no effect, but it appeared to add to the effect of the type-1 antagonist

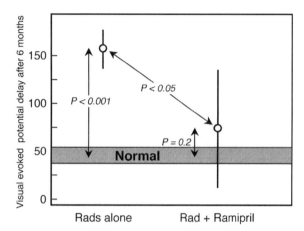

Fig. 9.7. Beneficial effect of the ACE inhibitor ramipril on experimental radiation neuropathy. A significant delay in the visual evoked potential tested at 6 months after irradiation occurs in rats undergoing 30 Gy irradiation of the optic nerves, and this delay is significantly shortened in rats that received ramipril in the drinking water starting at 2 weeks after irradiation. (Data from [23])

BMT chemo-irradiation conditioning [24]. We have called this syndrome BMT nephropathy. The use of ACE inhibitors and angiotensin blockers in patients with chronic renal failure of any cause is well accepted in clinical nephrology [25]. Combining the laboratory data with the nephrological principles provides compelling justification for use of ACE inhibitors or angiotensin antagonists in subjects with BMT nephropathy or classical radiation nephropathy. We thus recommend their use [26]. In one case of radiation nephropathy occurring after kidney transplantation, we showed clear-cut arrest of loss of function by use of an angiotensin antagonist [27]. Others have shown similar beneficial effects with ACE inhibitors in therapy of BMT nephropathy [28].

The ensemble of clinical and pre-clinical data on ACE inhibitors has justified their use in a mitigation trial in subjects undergoing TBI-based BMT. We are comparing captopril to placebo in adults and children undergoing TBI-based BMT at our center. The protocol of this study is schematized in Figure 9.8. We have enrolled almost 60 subjects since 1998, and interim safety analyses have not shown adverse effects on survival or disease relapse rates. In a parallel cohort, consisting of the 85 subjects who were eligible for this study, but declined to participate in it, we have defined the occurrence of chronic renal failure and the BMT nephropathy syndrome. These subjects received 14 Gy TBI (in nine fractions) with 30% renal shielding. Seven subjects developed chronic renal failure of which four have the BMT nephropathy syndrome. In the entire group, the median baseline serum creatinine was initially 0.8 mg/dl and this rose to 1 mg/dl at 1 year ($p=0.005$). In a historical cohort of 32 subjects who had undergone BMT between 1985 and 1989, and received 14 Gy TBI without renal shielding, there were ten cases of BMT nephropathy and the median serum creatinine for this cohort rose from 0.8 mg/dl at baseline to 1.3 mg/dl at 1 year ($p=0.0002$). Thus, there appears to be a greater rise in serum creatinine and a greater occurrence of BMT nephropathy in the unshielded cohort. These data confirm our previous report of the benefit of partial renal shielding on BMT nephropathy, and they provide further support for the notion that BMT nephropathy is a form of radiation nephropathy [29].

The clinical and laboratory data on ACE inhibitors for radiation nephropathy, and the laboratory data on their use in radiation pneumopathy have prompted the Radiation Therapy Oncology Group (RTOG) to launch a phase-II trial of captopril to reduce normal lung injury in subjects undergoing radiation therapy for lung cancer (RTOG – 0123 [30]). In this study, it will be tested whether late radiation lung toxicity (pneumopathy) will be significantly reduced by the use of captopril compared to no drug. The maximum dose of captopril to be used is 50 mg thrice daily, which is a usual therapeutic dose. This study is underway, and has enrolled 77 patients to date.

9.6 Conclusions

It is now reasonable to affirm that at least some normal tissue radiation injuries are treatable and some may be mitigated. In the case of lung, brain, and kidney, these benefits are achieved with ACE inhibitors and/or A_{II} receptor blockers, which suggests an important role for the RAS for these three tissues. Nonetheless, radiation-induced activation of the RAS has not been found. That may suggest that normal activity of this system is deleterious in the irradiated subject, or that its antagonists have an alternative (as yet undiscovered) mode of action.

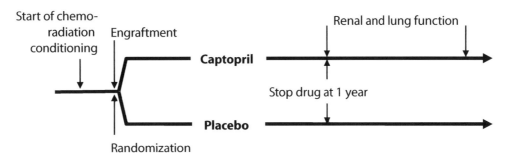

Fig. 9.8 Schema of the ongoing study of captopril to prevent chronic renal failure after BMT in adults and children undergoing TBI-based BMT at our center

Acknowledgements

Supported in part by NCI grant CA-24652 and NI-AID grant AI-067734. The human studies reported herein were approved by the Institutional Review Board of the Medical College of Wisconsin. The protocol for that analysis was written by Dr. Vasundhara Ganne.

References

1. Rubin P, Casarett GW (1968) Urinary tract: the kidney. In: Clinical radiation pathology, vol. 1. W.B. Saunders Co., Philadelphia, pp 293–333
2. Coleman CN, Stone HB, Moulder JE (2004) Modulation of radiation injury. Science 304:693–694
3. Moulder JE (2003) Pharmacological intervention to prevent or ameliorate chronic radiation injuries. Semin Radiat Oncol 13:73–84
4. Moulder JE (2004) Post-irradiation approaches to treatment of radiation injuries in the context of radiological terrorism and radiation accidents: a review. Int J Radiat Biol 80:3–10
5. Navar LG, Harrison-Bernard LM, Nishiyama A (2002) Regulation of intrarenal angiotensin II in hypertension. Hypertension 39:316–322
6. Ferreira SH, Bartelt DC, Greene LJ (1970) Isolation of bradykinin-potentiating peptides from Bothrops jararaca venom. Biochemistry 9:2583–2593
7. Lewis EJ, Hunsicker LG, Bain RP (1993) The effect of angiotensin-converting-enzyme inhibition on diabetic nephropathy. N Engl J Med 329:1456–1462
8. Moulder JE, Fish BL (1997) Angiotensin converting enzyme inhibitor captopril does not prevent acute gastrointestinal radiation damage in the rat. Rad Oncol Invest 5:50–53
9. Cohen EP, Lawton CA, Moulder JE (1993) Clinical course of late-onset bone marrow transplant nephropathy. Nephron 64:626–635
10. Moulder JE, Cohen EP, Fish BL (1993) Prophylaxis of bone marrow transplant nephropathy with captopril, an inhibitor of angiotensin-converting enzyme. Radiat Res 136:404–407
11. Cohen EP, Moulder JE, Fish BL (1994) Prophylaxis of experimental bone marrow transplant nephropathy. J Lab Clin Med 124:371–380
12. Moulder JE, Fish BL, Cohen EP (1997) Noncontinuous use of angiotensin converting enzyme inhibitors in the treatment of experimental bone marrow transplant nephropathy. Bone Marrow Transplant 19:729–736
13. Norman JT (1991) The role of angiotensin II in renal growth. Ren Physiol Biochem 14:175–185
14. Robbins MEC, Soranson JA, Wilson GD (1994) Radiation-induced changes in the kinetics of glomerular and tubular cells in the pig kidney. Radiat Res 138:107–113
15. Moulder JE, Fish BL, Regner KR (2002) Angiotensin II blockade reduces radiation-induced proliferation in experimental radiation nephropathy. Radiat Res 157:393–401
16. Moulder JE, Fish BL, Cohen EP (2002) Dietary sodium modification and experimental radiation nephropathy. Int J Radiat Biol 79:903–911
17. Cohen EP, Fish BL, Moulder JE (2002) The renin-angiotensin system in experimental radiation nephropathy. J Lab Clin Med 139:251–257
18. Moulder JE, Fish BL, Cohen EP (1998) Angiotensin II receptor antagonists in the treatment and prevention of radiation nephropathy. Int J Radiat Biol 73:415–421
19. Moulder JE, Fish BL, Cohen EP (1998) Brief pharmacologic intervention in experimental radiation nephropathy. Radiat Res 150:535–541
20. Siragy HM (2004) AT_1 and AT_2 receptor in the kidney: role in health and disease. Semin Nephrol 24:93–100
21. Ward WF, Lin PJ, Wong PS (1993) Radiation pneumonitis in rats and its modification by the angiotensin-converting enzyme inhibitor captopril evaluated by high-resolution computed tomography. Radiat Res 135:81–87
22. Ward WF, Molteni A, Ts'ao CH (1990) Captopril reduces collagen and mast cell accumulation in irradiated rat lung. Int J Radiat Oncol Biol Phys 19:1405–1409
23. Kim JH, Brown SL, Kolozsvary A (2004) Modification of radiation injury by Ramipril, inhibitor of angiotensin converting enzyme, on optic neuropathy in the rat. Radiat Res 161:137–142

24. Cohen EP, Lawton CA, Moulder JE (1995) Bone marrow transplant nephropathy: radiation nephritis revisited. Nephron 70:217–222
25. Cohen EP (2004) Chronic renal failure and dialysis. In Dale DC, Federman DD (eds) ACP Medicine. Web MD, New York
26. Cohen EP, Robbins MEC (2003) Radiation nephropathy. Semin Nephrol 23:486–499
27. Cohen EP, Hussain S, Moulder JE (2003) Successful treatment of radiation nephropathy with angiotensin II blockade. Int J Radiat Oncol Biol Phys 55:190–193
28. Antignac C, Gubler MC, Leverger G (1989) Delayed renal failure with extensive mesangiolysis following bone marrow transplantation. Kidney Int 35:1336–1344
29. Lawton CA, Cohen EP, Murray KJ (1997) Long-term results of selective renal shielding in patients undergoing total body irradiation in preparation for bone marrow transplantation. Bone Marrow Transplant 12:1069–1074
30. RTOG-0123 (2004) A Phase II randomized trial with captopril in patients who have received radiation therapy±chemotherapy for stage II-IIIB non-small cell lung cancer, stage I central non-small cell lung cancer, or limited-stage small cell lung cancer. Radiation Therapy Oncology Group, Philadelphia
31. Robbins MEC, Hopewell JW (1986) Physiological factors effecting renal radiation tolerance: a guide to the treatment of late effects. Br J Cancer 53[suppl VII]:265–267
32. Ward WF, Kim YT, Molteni A (1988) Radiation-induced pulmonary endothelial dysfunction in rats: modification by an inhibitor of angiotensin converting enzyme. Int J Radiat Oncol Biol Phys 15:135–140
33. Ward WF, Molteni A, Ts'ao CH (1989) Radiation-induced endothelial dysfunction and fibrosis in rat lung: modification by the angiotensin converting enzyme inhibitor CL242817. Radiat Res 117:342–350
34. Ward WF, Molteni A, Ts'ao C (1990) The effect of captopril on benign and malignant reactions in irradiated rat skin. Br J Radiol 63:349–354
35. Cohen EP, Fish BL, Moulder JE (1992) Treatment of radiation nephropathy with captopril. Radiat Res 132:346–350
36. Cohen EP, Lawton CA (1998) Pathogenesis, prevention and management of radiation nephropathy. In: Tobias JS, Thomas PRM (eds) Current radiation oncology. Oxford University Press, New York, pp 94–109
37. Molteni A, Moulder JE, Cohen EP (2000) Control of radiation-induced pneumopathy and lung fibrosis by angiotensin converting enzyme inhibitors and an angiotensin II type 1 receptor blocker. Int J Radiat Biol 76:523–532
38. Moulder JE, Fish BL, Cohen EP (2004) Impact of angiotensin II type 2 receptor blockade on experimental radiation nephropathy. Radiat Res 161:312–317

Second Malignancies as a Consequence of Radiation Therapy

Eric J. Hall and David J. Brenner

CONTENTS

10.1 Introduction 77
10.2 The Impact of IMRT on the Incidence of Radiation-Induced Second Cancers 79
10.3 Protons 81
10.4 The Bottom Line 81
References 81

10.1 Introduction

The use of radiation has such an established place in the practice of medicine, both for the diagnosis of multiple ailments and for the therapy of cancer, that it would be difficult to imagine modern medicine without X-rays. Each year worldwide, 2 billion diagnostic X-ray procedures are performed, while 5.5 million patients receive radiotherapy. With so many individuals exposed to an agent that is a known and proven human carcinogen, it is prudent to ask if there is a price tag.

It has been estimated that 10% of all patients presenting at major cancer centers in the US do so with a second malignancy. Second cancers arise from: (a) continued lifestyle, (b) genetic susceptibility, or they are (c) treatment-related. It is difficult to persuade individuals to change their life-style, and while individuals with a known genetic disorder may have an alarmingly high risk for second and even third malignancies, they account for a relatively small

E. J. Hall, DPhil, DSc, FACR, FRCR
D. J. Brenner, PhD, DSc
Center for Radiological Research, Columbia University Medical Center, College of Physicians & Surgeons, 630 W. 168th St, P&S 11-230, New York, NY 10032, USA

Summary

Radiation has an established place in the diagnosis and therapy of cancer. About 10% of patients presenting with cancer at major centers have a second malignancy. Most are a result of genetic predisposition or continued lifestyle, but some are treatment-related. For example, in patients treated for prostate cancer, about 1 in 70 develop a radiation-induced cancer by 10 years post therapy. Most second cancers are carcinomas arising in organs close to or remote from the treatment site. There is also an incidence of sarcomas within or close to the treatment volume, in the high dose region. The absolute risk is small, but the relative risk is high for these tumors. Animal studies show that the risk of a radiation-induced sarcoma approaches 100% following high doses in animals followed for a lifetime. This suggests that the reason for the low sarcoma risk in patients receiving radiotherapy for prostate cancer is their short life expectancy.

Innovations such as intensity modulated radiotherapy (IMRT), while improving local tumor control and reducing early morbidity, are likely to increase the incidence of second cancers due to additional leakage radiation during protracted treatments. Protons may alleviate the problem, but only if scanning beams are available.

fraction of human cancers. Here, we direct attention to radiation-induced second malignancies.

There are many single-institution studies in the literature involving radiotherapy for a variety of sites that conclude that there was no increase in second malignancies, although a more accurate assessment would have been that the studies had limited statistical power to detect a relatively small increased incidence of second malignancies induced by the treatment [6].

Most radiation oncologists who see a limited number of patients with any given type of tumor do not see second malignancies as a serious problem. There are the well-known exceptions, such as the significant incidence of breast cancer in young women receiving radiotherapy for Hodgkin's lymphoma [1, 7, 9], where the effect is too large to be missed. However, in most instances, it is difficult to get a reliable estimate for the incidence of second cancers following radiotherapy because a truly appropriate control group is not available. The two principal exceptions are carcinoma of the cervix in women and carcinoma of the prostate in men, since in both of these examples surgery and radiotherapy are alternative choices, and so the patients treated with surgery constitute the ideal control.

In the year 2000, through a collaborative project with the Radiation Epidemiological Branch of the National Cancer Institute, we completed the largest ever study of second malignancies in patients treated for prostate cancer. Data regarding the rate of incidence from the Surveillance, Epidemiology, and End Results (SEER) Program cancer registry (1973–1993) [2] were used to compare directly second malignancy risks in 51,584 men with prostate carcinoma who received radiotherapy (3549 of whom developed second malignancies) with 70,539 men who underwent surgery without radiotherapy (5055 of whom developed second malignancies). Data were stratified by latency periods, age at diagnosis, and site of the second malignancy.

Radiotherapy for prostate carcinoma was associated with a small, statistically significant increase in the risk of solid tumors relative to treatment with surgery. Among patients who survived for ≥5 years, the increased relative risk reached 15%, and was 34% for patients surviving ≥1 years (Fig. 10.1). The pattern of excess second malignancies among men treated with radiotherapy was consistent with radiobiologic principles in terms of site, dose, and latency. In absolute terms, 1 in 70 patients who received radiotherapy for prostate cancer will develop a second malignancy if they survive for 10 years following treatment.

A closer look at this study of prostate cancer patients reveals some interesting biologic insights. Analyzing the solid tumors site by site, there were significant radiation-associated increases in bladder carcinoma, rectal carcinoma, and lung carcinoma, as well as sarcomas in or near the treatment field. The distribution of second cancers is also shown in Fig. 10.1. It is interesting to note that the increase in relative risk for carcinoma of the lung, which was exposed to a relatively low dose (about 0.5 Gy), is of the same order as that for carcinomas of the bladder, rectum, and colon, all of which were subject to much higher doses (typically more than 5 Gy).

Although the larger number of radiation-associated malignancies clearly are carcinomas, as in the Japanese A-bomb survivors, the largest increase in relative risk is for in-field sarcomas, where it reaches over 200% at 10 years. This is a category of malig-

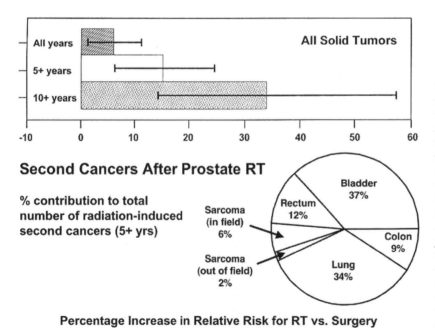

Fig. 10.1. The *upper panel* shows the percentage increase in relative risk for all solid tumors as a function of time after radiotherapy. The error bars represent 95% confidence limits. "*All years*" refer to all years post-treatment; the standard error is smaller in this case because of the larger number of patients; most did not survive to 5 or 10 years. The *lower panel* shows the distribution of the principal radiation-induced cancers, namely bladder, lung, rectum, and colon. There are also a small number of sarcomas that appear in heavily irradiated areas. (Data from [2])

nancy not observed in excess in the A-bomb survivors. In this, as in the majority of other studies, radiation-induced sarcomas occur only in heavily irradiated sites, close to the treatment volume. These observations most likely reflect a different mechanism for the induction of sarcomas compared with carcinomas. Carcinomas arise in tissues where, even in the adult, cells are turning over and/or are under hormonal control. By contrast, the target cells for sarcoma typically are dormant cells and large doses are needed to produce sufficient tissue damage to stimulate cellular proliferation. The sarcoma data in prostate patients appear to follow this pattern, with significant radiation-associated risks being observed for sites in and close to the treatment volume but not for more distant sites, which received lower doses.

The most probable reason that so few sarcomas were observed in the prostate patients is that most lived for such a short time after radiation therapy. A comparison with animal data is enlightening. A study at the National Institute of Health in the US involved irradiating Beagle dogs with large single doses in order to determine the tolerance of various organs in preparation for a program of intraoperative radiation therapy (IORT) [5]. An unexpected observation was that 25% of the dogs that received 25 Gy or more developed an in-field sarcoma with a latency of 3.6 years. This was an incidental observation, and not the purpose of the study. Dr. A. van der Kogel has irradiated a large number of rats in the study of radiation effects on the spinal cord. It was again an incidental observation that 50% of the animals who received 50 Gy developed a sarcoma, while 20% of those exposed to 20 Gy developed a sarcoma (A. van der Kogel, personal communication). Two decades ago, Herman Suit studied the incidence of radiation-induced sarcoma in defined flora and specific pathogen free mice, which had a life expectancy of 900–1000 days [8]. He showed that 50% of the animals developed a sarcoma by 480 days after a dose of 6.5–7.5 Gy, and 85% of the animals developed a sarcoma by 800 days. In comparing the animal data with the human experience, the latency periods must be thought of relative to the life span of the animals, i.e., the animals were observed for a much longer period post-irradiation relative to their life than were the radiotherapy patients, as illustrated in Fig. 10.2. The conclusion is that the incidence of sarcomas in heavily exposed tissues approaches 100% if a sufficiently long period is available for study following radiation.

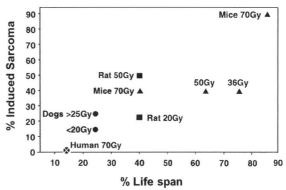

Fig. 10.2. Percent radiation-induced sarcomas as a function of time after irradiation, expressed as a percentage of normal life-span, for humans, dogs, rats, and mice. The number of sarcomas is also dependent on the radiation dose, but, in particular, it increases with time. The fact that radiation-induced sarcomas are rare in radiotherapy patients reflects the fact that most patients do not live for a large fraction of their life span after treatment

10.2
The Impact of IMRT on the Incidence of Radiation-Induced Second Cancers

The move from three-dimensional conformed radiotherapy (3D-CRT) to intensity-modulated radiation therapy (IMRT) involves more treatment fields. The dose-volume histograms (Fig. 10.3) show that, as a consequence, a larger volume of normal tissue is exposed to lower doses in the case of IMRT compared with 3D-CRT. In addition, the number of monitor units is increased by a factor of 2–3, increasing the total body exposure due to leakage radiation from the accelerator head. Both factors will tend to increase the risk of second cancers. Before an estimate can be made of the consequences of these two factors, we must arrive at a dose–response relationship for radiation-induced cancer. For single whole-body exposures, the relationship between mortality from solid tumors among the A-bomb survivors is consistent with linearity up to about 2.5 Sv. There is considerable uncertainty concerning the shape of the dose–response relationship for higher doses in the context of radiotherapy, where limited volumes of tissue receive doses of 20, 30, to even 70 Gy, while a much larger volume receives a lower dose because it is exposed to only some of the treatment fields.

Several possibilities can be entertained. First, it might be expected that the risk of inducing cancer

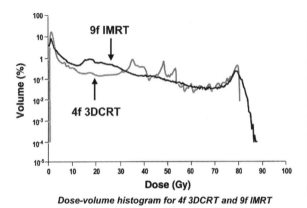

Fig. 10.3. Dose–volume histograms for two typical treatment plans for prostate cancer; a four-field conformal plan and a nine-field plan using intensity modulation. (From [4])

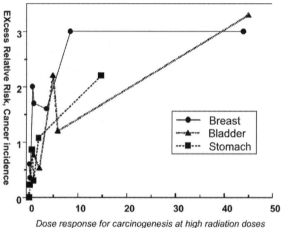

Fig. 10.4. Excess relative risk as a function of dose for three types of radiation-induced human solid cancers. The low-dose data came from the A-bomb survivors, while the high-dose data refer to radiotherapy patients. (Data compiled by Dr. Elaine Ron)

would fall off sharply at higher doses due to cell killing, on the grounds that dead cells cannot give rise to a malignancy. However, none of the dose–response curves for radiation-induced cancer in humans have this shape. It must be regarded, therefore, as an extreme possibility. The other extreme possibility, suggested by the data from some human studies, is that the risk of solid tumors shows a leveling off at 4–8 Gy with no decline thereafter. An intermediate case is represented by women who have been treated with radiation for cervical cancer and have an increased risk of developing leukemia, but the dose–response relationship is complex: the risk increases with doses up to about 4 Gy and decreases slowly at higher doses.

Figure 10.4 shows data for excess relative risk over a wide range of doses for three types of human cancers. The low-dose data came from the A-bomb survivors, and the high-dose data came from radiotherapy patients. It is quite evident that excess relative risk is not a linear function of dose, but rather it tends to plateau after rising steeply with dose up to about 5 Gy. These data imply that there is comparatively little change in relative risk from 5 to 50 Gy, so that in this range it is the volume of normal tissue exposed that dominates the magnitude of the risk.

A simple way to compare 3D-CRT and IMRT is to assume, as a first approximation, that the cancer risk associated with irradiating part of the trunk is directly proportional to the volume irradiated. By a comparison of dose volume histograms for 3D-CRT and IMRT, it was estimated that IMRT might increase the risk of radiation-induced carcinomas by perhaps 0.5% [4].

Delivery of a specified dose to the isocenter from a modulated field, delivered by either dynamic IMRT or the step and shoot method of IMRT, will, in general, require the accelerator to be energized for longer (hence more monitor units are needed) compared with delivering the same dose from an unmodulated field [10]. Some years ago, we made measurements of scattered and leakage radiation using an anthropomorphic "Randoman" phantom [3]. We used ionization chambers to measure the dose to a breast while a four-field technique was used to deliver a dose of 70 Gy to the cervix. Using a 6-MV LINAC, the breast dose was 0.25 Gy, while, with a 20-MV LINAC, the dose consisted of 0.5 Gy of X-rays plus a photoneutron component of about 1 cGy. We need only consider the data for the 6-MV LINAC, since higher energies are not usually used for IMRT. The breast dose of 0.25 Gy translates into a risk of radiation-induced cancer of about 0.5%, using a risk estimate of 2%. It is a sobering thought that, when a patient lies on the treatment couch under a modern Linac, in addition to the dose directed at the tumour, they receive a total body dose due to leakage radiation that equals the average dose received by the survivors of Hiroshima and Nagasaki. The total extra cancer risk posed by IMRT is the sum of that due to the extra volume of normal tissue exposed, (0.5%) and the total body dose due to extra leakage resulting from a doubling of the number of monitor units (0.5%); in other words, the change to IMRT results in about a doubling of the incidence of second cancers observed compared with more conventional radiation therapy.

10.3 Protons

Protons offer the possibility of reducing the volume of normal tissue involved, which one might expect to reduce the risk of second malignancies. However, for facilities where passive modulation is used (i.e., scattering foils), the total body neutron dose is likely to more than negate the gains from dose distribution. The use of a scanning beam greatly reduces the production of neutrons and in this situation the full potential advantage of protons can be realized.

10.4 The Bottom Line

In Western countries, rather more than half of all cancer patients receive radiotherapy at some stage in the management of their disease. Because of the latent period between exposures to radiation and the appearance of a radiation-induced cancer, studies show that the incidence of second malignancies following radiotherapy increases with time after treatment. In older patients that survive 10 years, about 1.5% will develop a radiation-induced second cancer. This percentage is likely to be approximately doubled by new sophisticated techniques, such as IMRT, which deliver a higher curative dose to the primary cancer, but result in more radiation to adjacent organs and to the whole body.

Second cancers become an increasing problem as treatment techniques improve, since patients must survive the first cancer in order to develop a second. It also becomes more of a problem as younger patients become candidates for radiotherapy. Protons may alleviate the problem, but only if scanning beams are available.

Acknowledgements

This research was supported in part by the Office of Science (BER), U.S. Dept of Energy Grant No. DE-FG02-03ER63629, and by a grant from NASA NAG 9-1519.

References

1. Bhatia S, Robison LL, Oberlin O (1996) Breast cancer and other second neoplasms after childhood Hodgkin's Disease. N Engl J Med 334:745–751
2. Brenner DJ, Curtis RE, Hall EJ (2000) Second malignancies in prostate carcinoma patients after radiotherapy compared with surgery. Cancer 88:398–406
3. Hall EJ, Martin SG, Amols H (1995) Photoneutrons from medical linear accelerators – radiobiological measurements and risk estimates. Int J Radiat Onc Biol Phys 33:225–230
4. Hall EJ, Wuu, CS (2003) Radiation-induced second cancers: the impact of 3D-CRT and IMRT. Int J Radiat Onc Biol Phys 56:83–88
5. Johnstone PAS, Laskin WB, DeLuca AM (1996) Tumors in dogs exposed to experimental intraoperative radiotherapy. Int J Rad Onc Biol Phys 34:853–857
6. Movas B, Hanlon AL, Pinover W (1998) Is there an increased risk of second primaries following prostate irradiation? Int J Rad Oncol Biol Phys 41:251–255
7. Nyandoto P, Muhonen T, Joensuu H (1998) Second cancers among long-term survivors from Hodgkin's Disease. Int J Radia Oncol Biol Phys 42:373–378
8. Suit HD, Sedlacek R, Fagundes L (1978) Time distributions of recurrences of immunogenic and nonimmunogenic tumors following local irradiation. Radiat Res 73:251–266
9. Travis LV, Curtis RE, Boice JD Jr (1996) Late effects of treatment for childhood Hodgkin's Disease. N Engl J Med 335:352–353
10. Williams PC, Hounsell AR (2001) X-ray leakage considerations for IMRT. Br J Radiol 74:98–102

Using Quality of Life Information to Rationally Incorporate Normal Tissue Effects into Treatment Plan Evaluation and Scoring

Moyed Miften, Olivier Gayou, David S. Parda, Robert Prosnitz, and Lawrence B. Marks

CONTENTS

11.1 Introduction 84
11.2 Methods 84
11.2.1 Theory 84
11.2.2 Treatment Plan Evaluation 85
11.2.2.1 Comparing Lung Plans for a Single Patient 85
11.2.2.2 Comparing Lung Treatment Plans from a Group of Patients 86
11.3 Results and Discussion 86
11.4 Conclusions 89
References 89

Summary

Sophisticated planning systems now readily provide the treatment planner with an increasing number of competing treatment plans. There is, however, no generally accepted method to compare and rank these competing treatment plans. A "realistic" approach utilizing decision analysis tools to rank treatment plans based on quality adjusted life years (QALY) expectancy was developed. The decision analysis methods were applied to the concept of uncomplicated tumor control probability (UTCP). The expected outcome for an anticipated course of radiation was described as a series of probabilities: alive, free of disease without complication; alive with disease; alive with complication, etc. For each of these states of health, a utility can be assigned based on published work or empirical estimates. The total QALYs for a particular treatment plan represent the product of duration-weighted states of health. The formalism for UTCP was generalized to incorporate the total QALY ($UTCP_{QALY}$) for a particular treatment. This approach was applied to compare competing treatment plans for a patient receiving high-dose external beam irradiation for unresectable non-small cell lung cancer. The plan ranking based on the traditional UTCP and QALY-weighted UTCP ($UTCP_{QALY}$) values was different. The QALY-weighted UTCP better reflects the importance of tumor control over mild complication, by giving less weight to the latter. This was confirmed by applying the method to clinical data from 201 lung cancer patients, 39 of whom developed radiation-induced pneumonitis (RP). The construct presented represents a potential improvement in the current methods used to compare competing treatment plans. Formulas presented are straightforward and can be readily incorporated into treatment planning systems.

M. Miften, PhD
Department of Radiation Oncology, Allegheny General Hospital, Associate Professor, Drexel University College of Medicine, 20 East North Avenue, Pittsburgh, Pennsylvania 15212, USA
O. Gayou, PhD
Department of Radiation Oncology, Allegheny General Hospital, Assistant Professor, Drexel University College of Medicine, 320 East North Avenue, Pittsburgh, Pennsylvania 15212, USA
D. S. Parda, MD
Department of Radiation Oncology, Allegheny General Hospital, Associate Professor, Drexel University College of Medicine, 320 East North Avenue, Pittsburgh, Pennsylvania 15212, USA
R. Prosnitz, MD
Assistant Professor, Department of Radiation Oncology, Duke University Medical Center, P.O. Box 3085, Durham, North Carolina 27710, USA
L. B. Marks, MD
Professor, Department of Radiation Oncology, Duke University Medical Center, P.O. Box 3085, Durham, North Carolina 27710, USA

11.1 Introduction

Modern radiotherapy treatment planning systems provide an increasing number of competing treatment plans. For most clinical situations, a number of treatment plans will achieve a specific set of dose/volume objectives. The decision to select a particular plan for treatment is generally made by a radiation oncologist based on training and clinical experience. The criteria applied are often poorly-defined, qualitative, and largely based on clinical judgment, tradition, and familiarity.

Mathematical algorithms and dose-response models, based on statistical theories such as the tumor control probability (TCP) model and the normal tissue complication probability (NTCP) model, have been developed to better objectively quantify this decision process. While such models have been incorporated into planning systems to compare treatment plans, there is still, however, no generally accepted method to score and rank these competing treatment plans. The concept of "uncomplicated tumor control probability" (UTCP) has been used previously [1–4].

$$UTCP = TCP\,(1-NTCP) \tag{11.1}$$

However, this approach weights a complication equal to a tumor relapse and ignores severity/grades of complications, which is certainly not clinically realistic. For example, mild lung fibrosis is not nearly as important as transverse myelitis. Furthermore, a study by Langer et al. [5] reported that this score function should not be used to draw conclusions on treatment techniques without statements of errors in the TCP and NTCP values. A number of studies suggested the use of weighting coefficients in the UTCP score function to allow for differences in tissue importance and the use of critical elements architecture for calculating NTCPs [6, 7]. However, uncertainty in tissue weighting introduces additional errors/uncertainties in plan ranking with UTCP. It is often up to the treatment planner to weigh those elements according to personal priorities using a complex mix of emotion and logic. These concerns/shortcomings have limited the broad application of the UTCP concept in the plan-evaluation process. Thus, we do not presently have a rationale and/or objective/quantitative method to incorporate normal tissue concerns into the radiation treatment planning process.

The concepts of decision analysis tools and quality adjusted life years (QALY) have been used to compare different medical interventions [8–11]. Decision analysis tools may provide a more realistic approach to rank treatment plans based on QALY expectancy. We herein expand the UTCP formalism to include the concept of QALY using decision analysis methods to better quantify the treatment plan selection process. This approach is first applied to a case example, comparing four competing plans for a patient with unresectable non-small-cell lung cancer, and then to a set of 201 patients who were treated for lung cancer with external-beam radiotherapy, 39 of whom developed radiation-induced pneumonitis (RP).

11.2 Methods

11.2.1 Theory

The expected outcome for an anticipated course of radiation can be described as a series of probabilities for different states of health: alive, free of disease without complication; alive with disease; alive with complication, etc. For each of these states of health, a "utility value" can be assigned, based on published work or empirical estimates, (e.g., 0 = death; 1 = alive and normal; 0.8 = alive, but short of breath on oxygen). The utility value quantifies the relative quality of life for each state of health. For example, 20 days on oxygen may be considered worth 15 days alive without a complication.

This approach can be used to calculate a QALY-adjusted probability of non-complication in normal tissue, $(1-NTCP)_{QALY}$. For instance, the $NTCP_{QALY}$ for a single organ represents the product of utility-duration-weighted states of health (i.e., grades of toxicity).

$$\begin{aligned}(1-NTCP)_{QALY} = &[1-Duration_1 \cdot (1-Utility_1) \cdot NTCP_1] \cdot \\ &[1-Duration_2 \cdot (1-Utility_2) \cdot NTCP_2] \cdots\end{aligned} \tag{11.2}$$

Substituting Eq. 11.2 in 11.1, the conventional UTCP formalism of a treatment plan can be generalized by incorporating the QALY information as follows:

$$UTCP_{QALY} = TCP\,(1-NTCP)_{QALY} \qquad (11.3)$$

$$UTCP_{QALY} = TCP \underbrace{\prod_{i=1}^{N}[1- \underbrace{Duration_i}_{\text{Duration factor}} \cdot \underbrace{(1-Utility_i)}_{\text{Utility factor}} \cdot NTCP_i]}$$

where the index i indicates that the calculation is performed for all states of health in a complication (i.e., all grades of a complication). The duration factor is calculated by the ratio of the average duration of each state of health (i.e., complication grade) relative to the average patient life expectancy (duration/life-expectancy). The utility factor quantifies the relative quality of life for each state of health in complication. Note that Eq. 11.3 can be used for all critical structures at risk for complications.

The formalism above represents the classic UTCP formula, with utility-weighted, duration-weighted, and probability-weighted values for states of health in complications. The values can be derived from true patient-rated quality of life information, when available. This formalism can be readily expanded to the full QALY approach by incorporating health-state transition probabilities estimated from the literature and applying a Markov stochastic system approach.

11.2.2
Treatment Plan Evaluation

11.2.2.1
Comparing Lung Plans for a Single Patient

Several competing treatment plans, consisting of one traditional three-dimensional conformal radiotherapy (3DCRT) plan and three intensity-modulated radiotherapy (IMRT) plans, were generated from a patient that we treated with high-dose external beam irradiation for unresectable non-small-cell lung cancer. The structures of interest, such as gross target volume, clinical target volume, and normal structures were defined and segmented on multiple CT images.

The competing plans were generated using PLUNC treatment planning software (Plan UNC, University of North Carolina), all using 15-MV photons [12]. The 3DCRT plan used anterior-posterior opposed fields to 46 Gy with oblique off-cord "axial" boost fields. The boost field orientation was selected to provide acceptable coverage to the gross disease, yet minimize dose to the lung. The IMRT plans were generated with the goal of further sparing the critical structures beyond that achieved with the 3DCRT plan.

The different IMRT treatment plans resulted from the use of slightly different dose-volume optimization constraints. A uniform set of six coplanar fields was used for all IMRT plans. A dose prescription of 78 Gy to the 95% isodose line, which covers the target volume, was used for the 3DCRT and IMRT plans. Minimum and maximum doses of 98% and 103% relative to the prescription dose were used as the target dose-volume constraints. As a starting point, the critical structures' dose-volume constraints for the lung plans were defined based on the data of Emami et al. [13] and Burman et al. [14], respectively. The dose-volume constraints for critical structures are listed in Table 11.1. For each plan, TCP, NTCP, the traditional UTCP (Eq. 11.1), and utility-duration weighted UTCP ($UTCP_{QALY}$) (Eq. 11.3) values were computed. The grade distribution, utility, and duration factors, as well as the life expectancy values used, were the same as in the multi-patient study which is discussed in Sect. 11.2.2.2.

The TCP model used in this work is based on the principles of the linear-quadratic model of cell survival [15]. In the TCP model, a value of 0.35 Gy^{-1} was used for the mean radiosensitivity of a cell population (α_{mean}). The standard deviation (σ_α), or level of inter-patient variability of radiosensitivity, was set to 0.08 Gy^{-1}. A clonogenic cell density of 1.5 million/cc was assumed. The effective doubling time for tumor clonogens (T_{eff}) of 5 days was used in the lung plans. The overall elapsed time (T) of 39 days, over the course of radiotherapy treatment,

Table 11.1. The dose-volume constraints used for critical structures in the lung IMRT plans

Dose-volume constraints		
Structure	Dose (Gy)	Volume (%)
Lungs	20	30
	35	15
Heart	30	100
	40	66
	45	0
Esophagus	50	100
	60	33
	80	0
Spinal cord	45	0

was used. The time between the first treatment and when tumor proliferation begins (kick-off time, T_k) was set to 0.

The NTCP model parameters used in this study are based on the work of Burman et al. [14]: the volume dependence (n), NTCP versus dose slope (m), and the dose-to-reference volume leading to 50% complication (TD_{50}). The NTCP values for these patients were calculated using the following parameter values: $TD_{50} = 30.5$ Gy, $m = 0.3$ and $n = 1$. These parameter values were similar to the ones used in the multi-institutional study by Kwa et al. [16]. The exact models including the cell kinetics and other parameter values used to compute the TCP and NTCP, respectively, are not critical to the results, although the same values must be applied in each model for valid comparison. Similar results would be obtained with alternative models.

11.2.2.2
Comparing Lung Treatment Plans from a Group of Patients

Dose-volume histograms from 201 lung cancer patients treated with external-beam radiotherapy at Duke University Medical Center between 1991 and 1999 [17] were compared and ranked using the UTCP and UTCP$_{QALY}$ methods. Of the 201 patients 39 developed RP. For more details on patient demographics, dosimetry, and planning techniques, etc., the reader is referred to Hernando et al [17]. Based on the clinical outcome data of these lung cancer patients, we estimated that patients with pneumonitis would have a grade distribution of 10.3%, 69.2%, and 20.5% for grade 1, 2, and 3, respectively (grade 1 = shortness of breath, grade 2 = initiation or increase in steroids; grade 3 = initiation of oxygen; and grade 4 = ventilation or death) [17]. Utility values of 0.9, 0.8, and 0.3 were assigned for grade 1, grade 2, and grade 3 pneumonitis with an average duration of 1 month, 4 months, and 18 months, respectively. An average patient life expectancy of 20 months was used. The values were assigned based on our clinical experience [18, 19]. The exact selected values are not critical to illustrate the concept.

For each plan, the TCP, NTCP, UTCP, and UTCP$_{QALY}$ values were computed. The lung NTCP$_{QALY}$ adjusted for the overall rate of pneumonitis was calculated and used in Eq. 11.3, which is an overall lung NTCP score computed as the product of utility-duration weighted grades of pneumonitis.

11.3
Results and Discussion

Figure 11.1 shows the transverse dose distributions of the 3DCRT plan and one of the IMRT plans (IMRT-2) for the single patient study. Table 11.2 and Figure 11.2 show TCP, lung NTCP, UTCP, and UTCP$_{QALY}$ values for the 3D plan and the three IMRT plans. The 3DCRT plan has the highest TCP and the highest lung NTCP values, resulting in the lowest UTCP value. Compared with the 3DCRT plan, the IMRT plans were better in sparing the lung at the expense of losing some target coverage. The IMRT-2 plan has the lowest TCP and the lowest lung NTCP values that resulted in the lowest UTCP value among the IMRT plans. The conventional UTCP formalism scored IMRT-1 as the best plan. The UTCP$_{QALY}$ scoring ranks the 3DCRT plan as the best plan, reflecting the fact that it has the highest TCP. The spread of UTCP values is 1.7%, whereas the spread of UTCP$_{QALY}$ values is 5.0%, which is closer to the TCP spread of 6.0%.

The "classic" UTCP formula gives equal weight to the TCP and NTCP, which is reflected in the flatness of the UTCP curve in Figure 11.2. Since the different plans are designed to all be at the top of the typical bell-shaped UTCP curve, the variation in UTCP from one plan to another is small. However, it is generally accepted that since local tumor control is required to sustain life, it is always more important than non-life threatening mild normal tissue complication. Therefore, it is crucial to weight the NTCP by a factor that tends to decrease its importance, and more so for non-severe grades of complications than for very severe grades of complication. The probability for a severe complication is generally much smaller than for a lower grade of the complication, so they rarely play a role, but it is crucial that they be taken into account. This is illustrated in the case example: the 3DCRT plan has the highest TCP value; therefore, as complications are mild (mostly grade 2), it should be ranked highly, which is achieved by the UTCP$_{QALY}$ scoring, but not the UTCP scoring.

Figure 11.3 shows the TCP, NTCP, UTCP, and UTCP$_{QALY}$ data for 163 out of 201 patients treated with external beam radiotherapy. Figure 11.4 depicts the UTCP and UTCP$_{QALY}$ values for the patients with RP differentiated by complication grade. For the purpose of clarity of Figure 11.3, we kept only the 163 patients for whom the TCP was greater than 0.9; 33 out of these 163 patients developed RP. The fig-

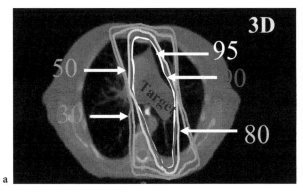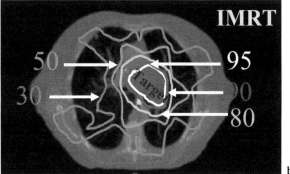

Fig. 11.1a,b. Percent relative isodose distributions for the 3DCRT plan (a) and IMRT-2 plan (b). The dose distributions show that the IMRT-2 plan is more conformal than the 3DCRT plan at the cost of slightly losing target coverage. Unlike the UTCP plan values, the UTCP$_{QALY}$ values, which incorporate clinically realistic quality of life data, suggest that the UTCP$_{QALY}$ formalism provides better differentiation between plans

Table 11.2. Tumor control probability (TCP) for the gross tumor volume, and normal tissue control probability (NTCP), for the lung of the 3DCRT and IMRT lung plans. Uncomplicated tumor control probability (UTCP) and pneumonitis QALY-weighted UTCP (UTCP$_{QALY}$) values for lung plans

Plan	Lung			
	TCP	NTCP	UTCP	UTCP$_{QALY}$ weighted for pneumonitis
3DCRT	90.8	6.8	84.6	89.8
IMRT-1	89.9	4.2	86.1	89.3
IMRT-2	85.4	0.6	84.9	85.3
IMRT-3	87.7	2.2	85.8	87.4

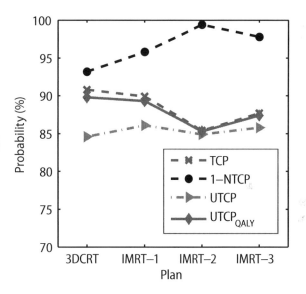

Fig. 11.2. TCP, 1-NTCP, UTCP, and UTCP$_{QALY}$ values for the 3DCRT and the three IMRT plans. The spread of UTCP$_{QALY}$ values of 5.0% is close to the TCP spread of 6.0%

ure shows that although the TCP values for all these patients were close to 1, the NTCP varied significantly. Consequently, the UTCP also varied significantly, reaching values of 0.5. Results in Figure 11.3 were ordered by decreasing UTCP. However, TCP and UTCP$_{QALY}$ were not monotonous functions of UTCP, explaining the noisy shape of their respective curve. The data in Figures 11.3 and 11.4 show that using UTCP$_{QALY}$ scoring, the mild complications' importance was downplayed significantly, with all UTCP$_{QALY}$ values above 0.83, thereby providing a more clinically realistic method for plan scoring. Note that a very small group of patients developed grade 3 pneumonitis and that no patient developed grade 4 pneumonitis, which is reflected in the high value of the UTCP$_{QALY}$ for all patients.

The traditional UTCP bell curve is shown in Figure 11.5. Theoretically, the best plan would be at the top of the curve. The effect of introducing the weighting in the UTCP$_{QALY}$ formalism is to modify this shape. The clinically relevant part of the curve is at its maximum or near the maximum. This happens at a higher dose for UTCP$_{QALY}$ than for UTCP, reflecting the fact that tumor control is more important than complication avoidance (i.e., the worst complication is uncontrolled tumor).

The usefulness of the UTCP$_{QALY}$ formalism depends on the incorporation of true patient-rated quality of life information and on the accuracy of the utility, complication grade duration, TCP, and NTCP values. The utility and duration values used in this work were estimated based on clinical expe-

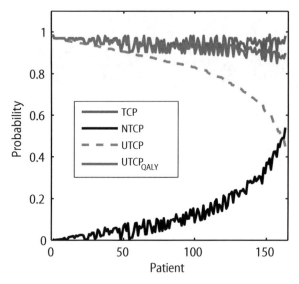

Fig. 11.3. TCP, NTCP, UTCP and UTCP$_{QALY}$ values for 163 lung cancer patients treated with external beam radiotherapy sorted in decreasing order of UTCP. Mild complications' importance is reduced with the UTCP$_{QALY}$ approach

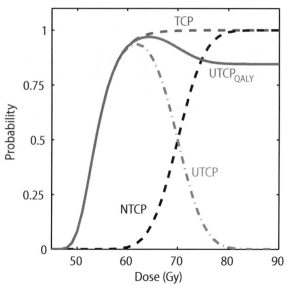

Fig. 11.5. Effect of the weight factors on the typical bell-shaped curve of UTCP as a function of delivered dose. The weight factors used to produce this curve are the ones used in the present study

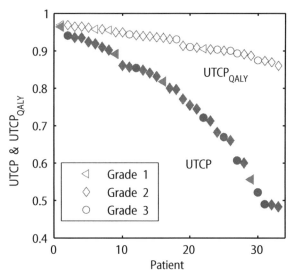

Fig. 11.4. UTCP$_{QALY}$ and UTCP distributions for different grades of pneumonitis observed in the 33 patients who developed the complication. Both distributions have been sorted independently in decreasing order

rience. Additional work is needed to better define these values. Large prospective studies are needed to better define the incidence of acute and late normal tissue risks. The utility values, and hence quality of life during times when experiencing a toxicity, need to be determined. The UTCP$_{QALY}$ approach affords a useful method to more rationally incorporate normal tissue risks into the planning process. The traditional UTCP method, that equally weights a complication with a tumor recurrence is not logical.

The examples shown in this article are intended only to present the mathematical and physical formulation of the UTCP$_{QALY}$ concept as well as its application. It can be readily expanded to include multiple organs. For example, the UTCP$_{QALY}$ approach can take into account the possibility that a patient develops several toxicities, each with their respective utility factors. However, this approach is not ideal. For example, it does not address the fact that the occurrences of different grades of the same complication are mutually exclusive of each other, i.e., one patient can not develop several grades of the same toxicity at the same time. No system will be able to definitively address all of the possible combinations of complications. However, if one can include most of the clinically important ones that impact quality of life or delivery of treatment and then summarize and assign the summary score among clinically important relative risk categories, this may provide enough utility in order to make choices among treatment options. Moreover, the ability to classify plans into different risk categories (low, medium, high, or extreme risk) may be clinically more relevant, especially when the dosimetric differences between plans are small.

It is important to stress that at the present stage the UTCP$_{QALY}$ concept should not be considered as a validated clinical model. The concept needs further development and refinements for clinical applications, such as radiotherapy treatments combined with chemotherapy.

11.4 Conclusions

A method utilizing decision analysis tools to rank treatment plans based on QALY expectancy was developed. The construct represents a potential improvement in the current methods used to compare competing treatment plans. The approach incorporates the probability of complication, the duration of particular states of health associated with the complication, as well as utilities for the time that the patient must spend in these altered states of health. Formulas presented are straightforward and can be readily incorporated into treatment planning systems.

Acknowledgments

This work was partially supported by NIH grant 69579 and Varian Medical Systems.

References

1. Kutcher GJ, Burman C, Brewster L et al (1991) Histogram reduction method for calculating complication probabilities for three-dimensional treatment planning evaluations. Int J Radiat Oncol Biol Phys 21:137–146
2. Leibel SA, Kutcher GJ, Harrison LB et al (1991) Improved dose distributions for 3D conformal boost treatments in carcinoma of the nasopharynx. Int J Radiat Oncol Biol Phys 20:823–833
3. Niemierko A, Urie M, Goitein M (1992) Optimization of 3D radiation therapy with both physical and biological end points and constraints. Int J Radiat Oncol Biol Phys 23:99–108
4. Photon Treatment Planning Collaborative Working Group (1991) State-of-the-art of external photon beam radiation treatment planning. Int J Radiat Oncol Biol Phys 21:9–23
5. Langer M, Morrill SS, Lane R (1998) A test of the claim that plan rankings are determined by relative complication and tumor-control probabilities. Int J Radiat Oncol Biol Phys 41:451–457
6. Jain NL, Kahn MG, Drzymala RE et al (1993) Objective evaluation of 3-D radiation treatment plans: a decision-analytic tool incorporating treatment preferences of radiation oncologists. Int J Radiat Oncol Biol Phys 26:321–333
7. Niemierko A, Goitein M (1991) Calculation of normal tissue complication probability and dose-volume histogram reduction schemes for tissues with a critical element architecture. Radiother Oncol 20:166–176
8. Hollen PJ, Gralla RJ, Kris MG et al (1993) Measurement of quality of life in patients with lung cancer in multicenter trials of new therapies. Cancer 73:2087–2098
9. Rotman M, Johnson DJ, Wasserman TH (2004) Supportive care and quality of life in radiation oncology. In: Perez CA, Brady LW, Halperin EC, Schmidt-Ullrich RK (eds) Principles and practice of radiation oncology. Lippincott, Philadelphia, pp 2426–2441
10. Kaplan RM (1993) Quality of life assessment for cost/utility studies in cancer. Cancer Treat Rev 19:85–96
11. Loomes G, McKenzie L (1989) The use of QALYs in health care decision making. Soc Sci Med 28:299–308
12. Chang SX, Cullip TG, Rosenman JG et al (2002) Dose optimization via index-dose gradient minimization. Med Phys 29:1130–1142
13. Emami B, Lyman J, Brown A et al (1991) Tolerance of normal tissue to therapeutic irradiation. Int J Radiat Oncol Biol Phys 21:109–122
14. Burman C, Kutcher GJ, Emami B et al (1991) Fitting of normal tissue tolerance data to an analytic function. Int J Radiat Oncol Biol Phys 21:123–135
15. Webb S, Nahum AE (1993) A model calculating tumor control probability in radiotherapy including the effects of inhomogeneous distributions of dose and clonogenic cell density. Phys Med Biol 38:653–666
16. Kwa SL, Lebesque JV, Theuws JC et al (1998) Radiation pneumonitis as a function of mean lung dose: an analysis of pooled data of 540 patients. Int J Radiat Oncol Biol Phys 42:1–9
17. Hernando ML, Marks LB, Bentel GC et al (2001) Radiation-induced pulmonary toxicity: a dose-volume histogram analysis in 201 patients with lung cancer. Int J Radiat Oncol Biol Phys 51:650–659
18. Etiz D, Marks LB, Zhou SM et al (2002) Influence of tumor volume on survival in patients irradiated for non-small-cell lung cancer. Int J Radia Oncol Biol Phys 53:835–846
19. Marks LB, Fan M, Clough R et al (2000) Radiation induced pulmonary injury: symptomatic verses subclinical endpoints. Int J Radiat Biology 76:469–475

Cancer-Related Fatigue as a Late Effect:
Severity in Relation to Diagnosis, Therapy, and Related Symptoms

Gary R. Morrow, Joseph A. Roscoe, Maralyn E. Kaufman, Christopher Bole, Colmar Figueroa-Moseley, Maarten Hofman, and Karen M. Mustian

12

CONTENTS

12.1 Introduction 92
12.2 **Methods and Materials** 92
12.2.1 Patients and Design 92
12.2.2 Measures 92
12.2.3 Statistical Analyses 93
12.3 **Results** 93
12.3.1 Research Participants 93
12.3.2 Severity of Symptoms 94
12.3.2.1 Severity Over Time by Treatment Type 94
12.3.2.2 Symptom Severity Remained Above Baseline After Therapy 94
12.3.2.3 Chemotherapy Patients Reported More Severe Symptoms than Those Receiving Radiation Alone 95
12.3.2.4 Patients Rated Fatigue As More Severe than Other Symptoms 95
12.3.3 Results for Radiation Alone Patients 95
12.3.3.1 No Differences in Fatigue Based on Age 95
12.3.3.2 Differences in Fatigue Based on Gender 96
12.3.3.3 Additional Subset Analyses 96
12.4 Discussion 96
References 98

G. R. Morrow, PhD, MS
Professor of Radiation Oncology, Professor of Psychiatry, Director, URCC-CCOP Research Base, Department of Radiation Oncology, James P. Wilmot Cancer Center, University of Rochester School of Medicine and Dentistry, Behavioral Medicine Unit, Box 704, 601 Elmwood Ave., Rochester, NY 14642, USA
J. A. Roscoe, PhD
M. E. Kaufman, PhD
C. Bole, MA
C. Figueroa-Moseley, PhD, MPH
M. Hofman, MS
K. M. Mustian, PhD
Department of Radiation Oncology, Behavioral Medicine Unit, James P. Wilmot Cancer Center, University of Rochester School of Medicine and Dentistry, 601 Elmwood Avenue, Box 704, Rochester, NY 14642, USA

Summary

Cancer-related fatigue (CRF) is widely recognized as the most distressing adverse effect experienced by cancer patients. We report on a large prospective survey conducted in part to characterize CRF severity in relation to depression and shortness of breath and to compare symptom severity in radiation and chemotherapy patients and over time. Careful characterization of CRF will aid in the development of effective methods to manage this disabling symptom.

A total of 776 patients completed a symptom inventory questionnaire before, during, and 6 months after the initiation of chemotherapy and/or radiation. Results were assessed by ANOVA, ANCOVA, and paired t-tests ($\alpha = 0.05$).

Fatigue was the most severe symptom in both therapy groups and 25% higher in women than men. The patterns over time for all three symptoms were similar (lowest at pre-treatment, significantly increased during treatment, and decreased at post-treatment, but remained significantly higher than pretreatment levels). For all symptoms and times, symptom severity was significantly greater in chemotherapy than radiation patients. This difference was confirmed in a breast cancer patient population.

We concluded that fatigue is the worst symptom in both therapy groups and worse for women than men. Overall, symptom severity was worse in chemotherapy than radiation patients and followed a distinct pattern over time. Symptom severity at 6 months post treatment remained elevated compared with baseline. These results suggest that treatment type and gender may be helpful in predicting and possibly managing the cluster of symptoms including CRF, depression, and shortness of breath.

12.1 Introduction

Fatigue is widely recognized as the most distressing of the multiple adverse effects experienced by patients with cancer before, during, and after receiving radiation therapy and/or chemotherapy [1–8]. Our research group has conducted two large prospective surveys of patients about to begin treatment for cancer, in part to help characterize CRF.

The first of these surveys [9] characterized the frequency, severity, course, and potential correlates of fatigue experienced by 372 patients with a variety of cancer diagnoses who were receiving radiation therapy without concurrent chemotherapy. These patients rated the presence and severity of each symptom on an 11-point scale of a symptom inventory (SI) once a week for 5 weeks. The results confirm that fatigue increases over time of treatment and that cancer type correlates with fatigue severity. At baseline (before treatment), 57% of the patients indicated they were fatigued. The percentage of the patient sample reporting fatigue significantly increased to 76% at week 3 ($p<0.001$) and then rose slightly to 78% at week 5. The mean severity of fatigue also increased significantly from a level of 1.9 at baseline to 2.6 at week 5 (37% increase; $p<0.001$). The proportion of patients who rated their fatigue as ≥4 also rose significantly ($p<0.001$), from 22% at baseline to 30% at week 5. The type of cancer accounted for 6.6%–9.5% of the variance in the severity of the fatigue at the five assessment times and was also a predictor of the symptom severity. From baseline to the fifth week of treatment, the frequency of fatigue increased for patients with prostate cancer (42%–71%), breast cancer (57%–77%), head and neck cancer (64%–93%), alimentary carcinoma (78%–87%), cancer of the nervous system (74%–85%), and lung cancer (78%–93%). After controlling for cancer type, neither gender nor age was predictive of fatigue severity at any time point.

The second prospective survey, reported herein, uses the same SI tool in a large population of cancer patients to compare the severity of fatigue to that of the related symptoms of depression and shortness of breath. In addition, symptom severity in patients receiving radiation therapy is compared with that in patients receiving chemotherapy. Thirdly, symptom severity is examined not only prior to and during therapy, but also 6 months following the conclusion of treatments. The objective of this study is to further characterize CRF in an effort to identify variables that would help in predicting and possibly managing CRF.

12.2 Methods and Materials

12.2.1 Patients and Design

Data were collected as part of a longitudinal study, funded by the National Cancer Institute (NCI), to assess the informational needs of cancer patients undergoing chemotherapy or radiation therapy. Several other articles have been published on different aspects of these data to date [10–12]. Participants were outpatients recruited from 17 private medical oncology practices throughout the US who were grantees of the NCI's Community Clinical Oncology Program (CCOP) and were members of the University of Rochester Cancer Center (URCC) CCOP Research Base between January 30, 2001 and September 13, 2002. Patients with diagnoses of breast, lung, prostate, hematologic, gastrointestinal, or head and neck malignancies were accrued to the study prior to their first treatment. Those who had prior chemotherapy or radiation therapy were not eligible, but those with prior surgery were eligible to enroll in the study. Demographic data, clinical diagnosis, and other pertinent patient information were obtained from the patients' medical records. All patients provided written informed consent prior to data collection, and the study was approved by the University of Rochester Human Research Subjects Review Board and the Internal Review Boards of the CCOPs.

12.2.2 Measures

Symptoms were assessed with the URCC symptom inventory (SI). This SI was modified from a clinical symptom checklist developed at the M.D. Anderson Cancer Center [13]. The SI is used by the patient to rate the presence and severity of each symptom on an 11-point horizontal scale ranging from 0 (not present) to 10 (as bad as you can imagine). The 12 symptoms that were assessed were fatigue, hair loss, difficulty concentrating, memory loss, nausea, hot flashes, depression, skin problems, sleep disturbances, pain, weight loss, skin problems, and shortness of breath. The SI is a useful, one-page questionnaire that is relatively simple to complete. Symptom severity was assessed before initiation of chemotherapy/radiation, during treatment, and 6 months after the completion of treatment.

12.2.3
Statistical Analyses

Pre-treatment symptom severity levels were compared to levels both during treatment and post-treatment using paired t-tests. Comparisons between/among subgroups of patients were made using t-test for independent samples and/or ANOVA, as appropriate. Additional analyses used analysis of co-variance (ANCOVA), controlling for age and type of treatment. The level of significance for all tests was set at $\alpha = 0.05$.

12.3
Results

12.3.1
Research Participants

Data from a total of 776 patients with a Karnosky performance index of at least 60 who completed a baseline SI and at least one subsequent SI assessment were analyzed. The demographic and clinical characteristics of the study population are shown by treatment type in Table 12.1. Overall, most patients were Caucasian, more than half had some college education, and most were married. An equal percentage (37%) of the patients received chemotherapy alone or radiation therapy alone, 25% of the study population received both types of treatments. More than half (65%) of the evaluable patients were female who were, on average, more than 8 years younger (mean, 58 years; range, 22–88 years) than the male patients (mean, 66 years; range, 20–92 years). The mean age of the patients who received radiation alone (65 years) was significantly higher ($p < 0.05$) than that of patients who received chemotherapy alone (58 years). Approximately 50% of the patients had breast cancer, about 20% had cancer of the genitourinary tract (typically prostate cancer), and about 10% had lung cancer. The radiation alone

Table 12.1. Demographic and clinical characteristics at baseline by therapy type

Characteristic	Chemotherapy alone $n = 289$	Radiation alone $n = 290$	Both $n = 197$
Age			
Mean (SD), (years)	58.1 (12.5)[a]	65.3 (11.2)[a,b]	57.1 (13.3)[b]
Range (years)	20–85	27–88	29–92
Sex			
Male	75 (26%)[a]	144 (50%)[a,b]	49 (25%)[b]
Female	214 (74%)	146 (50%)	148 (75%)
Race			
White	274 (95%)	270 (93%)	184 (93%)
Black	10 (3%)	18 (6%)	8 (4%)
Other	5 (2%)	2 (1%)	5 (3%)
Education			
Some College	163 (56%)	172 (59%)	107 (54%)
High School or less	126 (44%)	118 (41%)	90 (46%)
Marital status			
Married	211 (73%)	210 (72%)	141 (72%)
Not married	78 (27%)	80 (28%)	56 (29%)
Karnofsky Performance Status			
Mean (SD)	92.4 (10.0)[a]	95.0 (8.9)[a]	93.5 (9.0)
Range	60–100	60–100	60–100
Primary cancer site			
Alimentary Tract	42 (14%)	2 (1%)	11 (6%)
Breast	153 (53%)	122 (42%)	125 (63%)
Genitourinary Tract	13 (4%)	125 (43%)	5 (2%)
Gynecologic	19 (7%)	14 (5%)	7 (4%)
Hematologic	34 (12%)	7 (2%)	8 (4%)
Lung	26 (9%)	15 (5%)	36 (18%)
Other	1 (0%)	7 (2%)	8 (4%)
Previous surgery	231 (80%)[a]	204 (70%)[a]	145 (74%)
Symptom severity, mean (SD)			
Fatigue	2.7 (2.3)[a]	1.9 (2.3)[a,b]	2.7 (2.7)[b]
Depression	2.3 (2.5)[a]	1.6 (2.4)[a,b]	2.4 (2.6)[b]
Shortness of Breath	1.2 (2.0)	0.9 (1.7)[b]	1.4 (2.3)[b]

[a,b] There was a significant difference between these groups ($p < 0.05$).

group had a higher proportion of genitourinary tract cancer patients (43%) than the chemotherapy group (7%). Because the symptom severity data for the three symptoms analyzed (i.e., fatigue, depression, and shortness of breath) did not significantly differ between the chemotherapy alone (without radiation therapy) group and the chemotherapy with radiation therapy group at any time point for any symptom, we collapsed the data across these two treatment groups for clinical clarity. This combination yielded a group of 486 patients (63%) that is hereafter referred to as the chemotherapy group.

12.3.2
Severity of Symptoms

The severity over time of three health-related characteristics from the SI (fatigue, depression, shortness of breath) in patients receiving chemotherapy and those receiving radiation alone is shown in Figure 12.1. Several patterns are evident in these results.

12.3.2.1
Severity Over Time by Treatment Type

The severity patterns over time for all three symptoms for both therapy groups were similar; that is, symptom severity was lowest at the pre-treatment assessment, increased and peaked during treatment, and then decreased at post-treatment for both treatment groups (Fig. 12.1). As reported in Table 12.2, chemotherapy patients reported a statistically significant increase in the mean severity of fatigue from 2.74 at baseline to 6.82 during treatment ($p<0.001$). Fatigue levels from this high point then dropped significantly following treatment to a mean of 3.84 ($p<0.001$). Similarly, fatigue increased significantly in patients receiving only radiation therapy from a baseline mean of 1.93 to a during treatment peak of 4.21 ($p<0.001$) and then dropped significantly to a mean of 2.98 following treatment ($p<0.001$). The severity of depression followed a similar pattern of significantly increasing during treatment, regardless of treatment type, and then significantly decreasing from these peak levels following treatment (all, $p<0.01$). Shortness of breath also increased significantly during treatments in both treatment groups (both, $p<0.001$). The decrease in this symptom following treatment, however, was significant only in the patients receiving chemotherapy ($p<0.01$) and not in patients receiving radiation treatments alone ($p<0.50$).

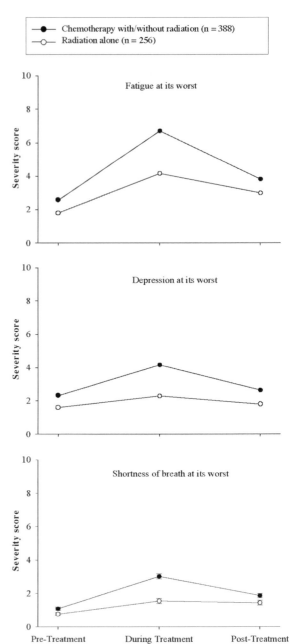

Fig. 12.1. Fatigue and associated symptoms over time in patients receiving chemotherapy and/or radiation treatments

12.3.2.2
Symptom Severity Remained Above Baseline After Therapy

Although the levels of symptom severity decreased by the post-treatment assessment, most remained significantly elevated compared with pre-treatment levels. This pattern was evident among both groups of patients, with one exception. Patients receiving ra-

Table 12.2. Comparison of mean (SE) symptom severity between radiation and chemotherapy patients

Symptom by assessment Period	Chemotherapy $n = 357$	Radiation $n = 238$	p-Value of t-test
Fatigue			
Baseline	2.59 (0.13)	1.80 (0.14)	(.000)
During treatment	6.70 (0.13)	4.16 (0.19)	(.000)
Post treatment	3.81 (0.15)	2.97 (0.18)	(.000)
Depression			
Baseline	2.33 (0.13)	1.61 (0.15)	(.000)
During treatment	4.17 (0.16)	2.29 (0.19)	(.000)
Post treatment	2.64 (0.16)	1.81 (0.17)	(.000)
Shortness of breath			
Baseline	1.08 (0.11)	0.76 (0.10)	(.041)
During treatment	3.01 (0.16)	1.54 (0.15)	(.000)
Post treatment	1.86 (0.13)	1.44 (0.15)	(.034)

diation alone reported an average level of depression post-treatment that was not significantly different from that at baseline. Paired t-tests confirmed that, aside from this exception, the increases in symptom severity from pre-treatment to the post-treatment period were statistically significant (all, $p < 0.05$). Hence, although symptom severity improved significantly after therapy, average levels of severity at 6 months post-treatment remained significantly worse than that before treatment.

12.3.2.3
Chemotherapy Patients Reported More Severe Symptoms than Those Receiving Radiation Alone

For all three symptoms in Figure 12.1, patients who received chemotherapy reported greater severity of symptoms than patients who received radiation alone at all assessment points. Multiple independent t-tests comparing the two groups across each symptom and at each time period (pre-treatment, during treatment, and post-treatment) showed these differences to all be significant ($p < 0.05$; Table 12.2).

12.3.2.4
Patients Rated Fatigue As More Severe than Other Symptoms

Symptom severity was rated higher for fatigue than the other symptoms both during and following treat-

ments for both therapy types. For patients receiving radiation therapy, the average severity of fatigue was 4.16 during treatments and 2.97 following therapy. The next most severe symptom at both treatment times was depression with rating of 2.29 and 1.81 for the during and post periods, respectively. The pattern was similar for patients receiving chemotherapy with the average severity of fatigue being 6.7 during treatments and 3.81 following therapy. The next most severe symptom at both treatment times for these patients was still depression with ratings of 4.17 and 2.64 for the during and post periods, respectively. Another indication that fatigue was the most problematic symptom was the degree of change from baseline. On average (both patient therapy groups combined), the severity of fatigue increased 139% from pre-treatment to the assessment during treatment, whereas the average severity of the other symptoms increased 90% during the same time period.

12.3.3
Results for Radiation Alone Patients

12.3.3.1
No Differences in Fatigue Based on Age

Independent t-tests showed no significant difference in levels of fatigue based on age, at any time point studied, using a median split at 67 years old (Fig. 12.2).

12.3.3.2
Differences in Fatigue Based on Gender

Independent *t*-tests showed significant differences in levels of fatigue based on gender in patients receiving radiation treatments (Fig. 12.3). The level of fatigue among women was statistically higher ($p<0.05$) than for men at baseline (2.14 and 1.48, respectively), during treatment (4.65 and 3.68, respectively), and following treatment (3.17 and 2.78, respectively), with the average level of fatigue across all three assessment times being 25% higher for women than for men.

12.3.3.3
Additional Subset Analyses

Subset analyses were conducted using only the 374 female breast cancer patients, the largest homogenous group of patients in the sample, to add clarity by controlling for gender and disease type in the fatigue severity comparisons. Women in both the chemotherapy and radiation therapy groups reported significant ($p \leq 0.001$) increases from baseline to during treatment (2.43 to 6.97 and 2.26 to 4.54, respectively) in the severity of fatigue (Fig. 12.4). In addition, the difference in fatigue severity between the two therapy groups at the during treatment assessment was statistically significant (6.97 vs. 4.54, $p<0.001$). No significant differences in the severity of fatigue between the chemotherapy and the radiation groups were noted at baseline or post-treatment. These findings were further supported by three tests using one-way ANOVA, controlling for patient age, which showed a significant difference between the two groups during treatment ($p<0.001$), but not at baseline or post-treatment (both, $p>0.30$).

12.4
Discussion

The SI results of this large, multicenter study of cancer patients receiving either chemotherapy or radiation therapy alone provide further characterization of the debilitating, prevalent side effects of cancer and its treatment. Overall, the results indicate that

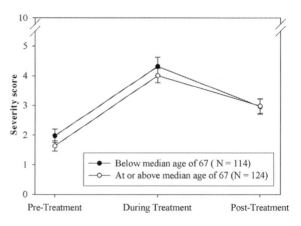

Fig. 12.2. Fatigue patterns over time in patients receiving radiation therapy by age

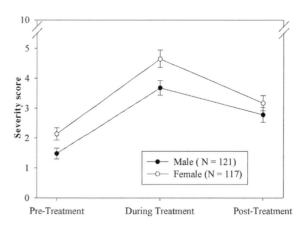

Fig. 12.3. Fatigue patterns over time in patients receiving radiation therapy by gender

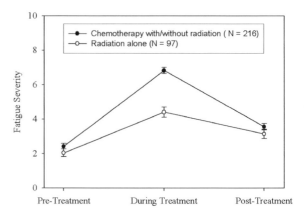

Fig. 12.4. Fatigue patterns over time in breast cancer patients by treatment type

the severity of fatigue is higher than that of depression and shortness of breath in both patient therapy groups at all times studied and higher in women than men. However, the pattern of fatigue severity over time is similar to that of the other symptoms in each therapy group (Fig. 12.1) and in men and women (Fig. 12.3). Although the time course of symptom severity is similar between therapy groups, there is a significantly greater overall severity of each of the three symptoms studied as reported by patients in the chemotherapy group compared with that reported by patients receiving radiation therapy alone (Fig. 12.1).

The observation that fatigue was rated as the most severe in our large patient sample parallels the abundant literature describing CRF as the most distressing symptom of cancer and its treatment [1–3, 5–8, 14, 15]. Depression was rated as the next most severe symptom by the two therapy groups. Depression is also common and disruptive in cancer patients [16–18]. Shortness of breath was the least severe of the three symptoms. Symptom severity for each symptom and each therapy group was lowest at the pre-treatment assessment, peaked during therapy, and decreased towards pre-treatment severity at 6 months post-treatment. A similar pattern of fatigue severity over time was also noted in both men and women receiving radiation therapy (Fig. 12.3).

The difference noted at baseline between the two therapy groups in symptom severity may be due in part to the substantially higher proportion of genitourinary tract cancer patients in the radiation alone group (43%) compared with the chemotherapy group (7%). Indeed, when gender and cancer type are controlled, there is no baseline difference between therapy groups for the symptom of fatigue (Fig. 12.4).

Although symptom severity improved significantly 6 months after therapy, post-treatment symptom severity remained significantly worse than pre-treatment levels for each symptom in each therapy group, with the exception of depression in radiation therapy patients. Results in the literature regarding symptom severity post treatment vary depending on multiple factors, including the symptom, study population, therapy regimen, assessment technique, etc. For example, in contrast to our findings, fatigue severity was reported to return to baseline within 3 months following radiation therapy in breast cancer patients [19] and following chemotherapy in patients with a variety of cancer types [20]. However, our results are similar to several studies [21–23], including that of Ahlberg et al. [1] who reported that increases in fatigue, loss of appetite, nausea/vomiting, and diarrhea persisted for 2–3 weeks post radiation therapy in patients with uterine cancer. The lingering effect of cancer therapy on patient fatigue, depression, and shortness of breath emphasizes the persistent suffering of cancer patient and the need to determine therapeutic management of debilitating side effects of treatment that may have an impact on patient compliance and survival [24].

Further analysis of the fatigue symptom in the radiation therapy group revealed that there were no differences based on age, but that women reported a 25% greater severity of this symptom than did men. As with many of the side effects of cancer-treatment-related side effects, the literature contains inconsistent results with regard to gender differences [25]. The presence or absence of gender differences in symptomatology related to cancer therapy depends on the typical variables of cancer type and stage, treatment type and duration, assessment technique, etc. This inconsistency confirms the need for individualized treatment of patients and further research in these complex symptoms.

Finally, our results show a clear distinction in severity of all symptoms between the two therapy groups. The overall severity of each of the three symptoms studied was reported as greater by patients in the chemotherapy group than those patients receiving radiation therapy alone. This significant distinction between symptom severities in the two therapy groups was noted in the entire, heterogeneous patient population (Fig. 12.1, Table 12.2) and verified for fatigue in the gender-, treatment type-, and disease type-controlled population of breast cancer patients receiving radiation (Fig. 12.4). Variations in symptom severity based on type of chemotherapy have been noted previously for fatigue [26, 27]. In a recent report on CRF in patients receiving chemotherapy and radiation, the authors discuss the results of five studies in which CRF was assessed in patients with a variety of cancer diagnoses [20]. In this report, CRF due to chemotherapy reached a peak 2–5 days after each chemotherapy session, remained elevated the week after each cycle of chemotherapy, and never returned to baseline. CRF due to radiation gradually accumulated over the course of the treatment but returned to near baseline values within 5 days of completing treatment. These results are similar to ours for fatigue, depression, and shortness of breath following chemotherapy, but differ from ours in the radiation therapy group.

These differences contribute to the conclusion that there are still inconsistencies in the characterization CRF and other cancer-treatment-related symptoms that need to be clarified.

In summary, the results of our study have the advantages of being from a prospective survey of a large patient population and that trends in a heterogeneous population (Fig. 12.1) were verified in an analysis that was controlled for cancer and treatment types (Fig. 12.4). We were able to show that fatigue is the worst of the symptoms studied in all therapy groups and worse for women than men. In addition, symptom severity was worse in patients receiving chemotherapy than those receiving radiation therapy. Finally, symptom severity followed a distinct and consistent pattern prior to, during therapy, and 6 months following the conclusion of both types of therapy. These results suggest that treatment type and gender may be helpful in predicting and possibly managing the cluster of symptoms including CRF, depression, and shortness of breath.

References

1. Ahlberg K, Ekman T, Gaston-Johansson F (2005) The experience of fatigue, other symptoms and global quality of life during radiotherapy for uterine cancer. Int J Nurs Studies 42:377–386
2. Ahlberg K, Ekman T, Gaston-Johansson F et al (2003) Assessment and management of cancer-related fatigue in adults. Lancet 362:640–650
3. Curt GA, Breitbart W, Cella D et al (2001) Impact of cancer-related fatigue on the lives of patients: new findings from the Fatigue Coalition. In: Marty M, Pecorelli S (eds) Fatigue and cancer, 1st ed. Elsevier, Amsterdam, pp 3–16
4. Irvine D, Vincent L, Graydon JE et al (1994) The prevalence and correlates of fatigue in patients receiving treatment with chemotherapy and radiotherapy. A comparison with the fatigue experienced by healthy individuals. Cancer Nurs 17:367–378
5. Morrow GR, Andrews PL, Hickok JT et al (2002) Fatigue associated with cancer and its treatment. Support Care Cancer 10:389–398
6. Morrow GR, Hickok JT, Lindke J et al (1999) Longitudinal assessment of fatigue in consecutive chemotherapy patients: an URCC CCOP study. Proc Annual Meeting Am Soc Clin Oncol 18:593a, (Abstract No. 2293)
7. Morrow GR, Shelke AR, Roscoe JA et al (2005) Management of cancer-related fatigue. Cancer Invest 23:225–235
8. Stasi R, Abriani L, Beccaglia P et al (2003) Cancer-related fatigue: evolving concepts in evaluation and treatment. Cancer 98:1786–1801
9. Hickok J, Roscoe J, Morrow GR et al (2005) Frequency, severity, clinical course and correlates of fatigue in 372 patients during five weeks of radiotherapy (RT) for cancer. Cancer 104:1772–1778
10. Hofman M, Morrow GR, Roscoe JA et al (2004) Cancer patients' expectations of experiencing treatment-related side effects: an University of Rochester Cancer Center – Community Clinical Oncology Program study of 938 patients from community practices. Cancer 101:851–857
11. Shields CG, Morrow GR, Griggs J et al (2004) Decision role preferences of patients receiving adjuvant cancer treatment: an University of Rochester Cancer Center Community Clinical Oncology Program. Supportive Cancer Ther 1:119–126
12. Yates JS, Mustian KM, Morrow GR et al (2005) Prevalence of complimentary and alternative medicine use in cancer patients during treatment. Support Care Cancer 13:806–811
13. Cleeland CS, Mendoza TR, Wang XS et al (2000) Assessing symptom distress in cancer patients: the M.D. Anderson Symptom Inventory. Cancer 89:1634–1646
14. Morrow GR, Roscoe JA, Bushunow P et al (2000) The relationship of circadian rhythm with fatigue and depression in breast cancer patients. Supportive Care Cancer 8:250
15. Vogelzang NJ, Breitbart W, Cella D et al (1997) Patient, caregiver, and oncologist perceptions of cancer-related fatigue: results of a tripart assessment survey. The Fatigue Coalition. Seminars Hematol 34:4–12
16. De Jong N, Candel MJJM, Schouten HC et al (2005) Course of mental fatigue and motivation in breast cancer patients receiving adjuvant chemotherapy. Annals Oncol 16:372–382
17. Hann D, Winter K, Jacobsen P (1999) Measurement of depressive symptoms in cancer patients: evaluation of the Center for Epidemiological Studies Depression Scale (CES-D). J Psychosom Res 46:437–443
18. Visser MR, Smets EM (1998) Fatigue, depression and quality of life in cancer patients: How are they related? Support Care Cancer 6:101–108
19. Irvine DM, Vincent L, Graydon JE et al (1998) Fatigue in women with breast cancer receiving radiation therapy. Cancer Nurs 21:127–135
20. Schwartz AL, Nail LM, Chen S et al (2000) Fatigue patterns observed in patients receiving chemotherapy and radiotherapy. Cancer Invest 18:11–19
21. Broeckel JA, Jacobsen PB, Horton J et al (1998) Characteristics and correlates of fatigue after adjuvant chemotherapy for breast cancer. J Clin Oncol 16:1689–1696
22. Loge JH, Abrahamsen AF, Kaasa S (2000) Fatigue and psychiatric morbidity among Hodgkin's disease survivors. J Pain Symptom Management 19:91–99
23. Smets EM, Visser MR, Willems-Groot AF et al (1998) Fatigue and radiotherapy: (A) experience in patients undergoing treatment. Br J Cancer 78:899–906
24. Scott HR, McMillan DC, Forrest LM et al (2002) The systematic inflammatory response, weight loss, performance status and survival in patients with inoperable non-small cell lung cancer. Br J Cancer 87:264–267
25. Miaskowski C (2004) Gender differences in pain, fatigue, and depression in patients with cancer. J Natl Cancer Inst Monogr 32:139–143
26. Berger A, Walker SN (2001) An explanatory model of fatigue in women receiving adjuvant breast cancer chemotherapy. Nurse Res 50:43–54
27. De Jong N, Candel MJJM, Schouten HC et al (2004) Prevalence and course of fatigue in breast cancer patients receiving adjuvant chemotherapy. Ann Oncol 15:896–905

Normal Tissue TNM Toxicity Taxonomy: Scoring the Adverse Effects of Cancer Treatment

Philip Rubin

CONTENTS

13.1 Introduction and Overview: Genesis and Evolution *100*

13.2 The Biologic Basis for Combining Acute and Late Criteria *101*

13.3 Validation, Standardization of Language, and Statistical Reporting *101*

13.4 Normal Tissue/Organ TNM Taxonomy for Adverse Effects of Cancer Treatment *103*
13.4.1 TNM Language *103*
13.4.2 General Rules *104*
13.4.3 New Definitions of TNM Applied to Adverse Effects of Normal Tissue *104*
13.4.4 Assigning the Grade for Progression *104*
13.4.5 Classification According to Evidence for Certainty of Grade *105*
13.4.6 Summary Toxicity Grade *105*
13.4.7 Global Toxicity Score of Multiple Organs *106*
13.4.8 Therapeutic Ratio Determination and Decision Making *106*

References *106*

Taxonomy and classification are attempts to order the chaos in nature

P. Rubin, MD
Professor and Chair Emeritus, Department of Radiation Oncology, former Associate Director of the James P. Wilmot Cancer Center, and former Associate in the Department of medicine and Surgery, University of Rochester School of Medicine and Dentistry, 601 Elmwood Avenue, Box 647, Rochester, NY 14642, USA

Summary

Philosophically, the TNM Cancer Classification is based on the premise that all malignant tumors have a similar life cycle. Cancers originate in a normal tissue, then spread regionally into lymph nodes and then to systematic distant sites hematogenously. In a parallel fashion, the conceptual design of a normal tissue TNM classification is based on a similarity of normal tissue injury following multimodal cancer treatment which is often greatest in the structure/organ of cancer origin and decreases in neighboring normal tissues. There may be a generalized or systemic toxicity.

$_NT$ = The normal Tissue, anatomic structure, organ in which the cancer arose and spreads initially.

$_NN$ = Neighboring or surrounding normal tissues or organs, viscera that are not involved by the tumor but in the regional nodal drainage zone.

$_NM$ = SysteMic effects that are generalized and include hematologic, hepatic toxicity, weight loss.

Longitudinal progression of an adverse effect can be designated numerically as the area under the curve of the "effect-time" course and becomes the operational taxonomic unit (OTU), i.e., the grade assigned is according to the criteria in CTCAE v3.0 or LENT/SOMA, or RTOG/EORTC which is 1+ Mild, 2+ Moderate, 3+ Severe, and 4+ life threatening. The translation of acute/late effect as subscripts to $_NT$ and $_NN$ allows for scoring of toxic effects over time of follow-up.

13.1 Introduction and Overview: Genesis and Evolution

Although dramatic improvements in cancer survival statistics have occurred over the past five decades and are well documented in the literature, the same has not been true for detailing the unwanted incidental adverse effects following multimodal cancer treatment. The dramatic gains in 5-year survival has been compiled by cancer site in a SEER tabulation marking the passing of 50% level for all cancers at the turn of this century [1]. At issue and unresolved is the price for the success and how to best measure and grade these adverse toxicity effects which persist and progress over time, detracting from the cancer survivor's quality of life.

The need for a grading system to assess treatment toxicities lagged behind the TNM classification of cancers. It was in the 1980s, because of the increasing number of clinical trials sponsored by the National Cancer Institute (NCI) and the European Organisation for Research on Treatment of Cancer (EORTC), that a consolidation of numerous individual approaches by each specialty was initiated. The genesis of acute toxicity scoring versus late effect grading originated in a bipolar fashion. The NCI Cancer Therapy Evaluation Program (CTEP) recognized the need to uniformly score the toxic acute and subacute effects of chemotherapy. The Common Toxicity Criteria (CTC), first published in 1983, were concerned with the physiologic and functional endpoints, many of which are transitory and reversible [2]. Then, version 2.0 attempted to incorporate the acute effects of other modalities such as radiation and expanded 13 to 22 organ systems and the number of criteria incremented from 18 to 260 (Table 13.1) [3].

The radiation oncology profession has traditionally been concerned with reporting late effects of cancer treatment and the Radiation Therapy Oncology Group (RTOG), in conjunction with EORTC, introduced both the "acute" and the "late" radiation morbidity scoring criteria simultaneously [4]. A series of NCI sponsored workshops led to the introduction of a more comprehensive system entitled: LENT ~ late effects normal tissue and SOMA criteria, representing subjective symptoms, objective findings and management features. The 'A' referred to analytic quantifiable parameters in the laboratory or imaging. With acceptance and joint publications on both sides of the Atlantic, RTOG/EORTC hoped to standardize reporting of late effects [5, 6]. Some of the guiding thoughts to reduce interobserver variability was to replace the commonly used four grades of 1+ mild, 2+ moderate, 3+ severe, 4+ life threatening with better descriptors with corresponding terms as occasional, intermittent, persistent and refractory, respectively, when referring to the expression of symptoms and signs, i.e., pain. Longitudinal clinical trials emphasizing correlation of symptoms and signs of toxicity with metrics and interventions are future goals [7].

The most recent collaboration sponsored by all modalities has resulted in a more comprehensive CTC v3.0, which includes more late effects criteria and is inclusive of all modalities [8, 9]. However, the merging of late effect and acute effect criteria, although more comprehensive with 510 criteria, when

Table 13.1. The evolution of toxicity grading systems (1979–1998)

System	No. of criteria	No. of organs	Modality	Phase
WHO (1979)	28	9	Chemo	Acute
CTC (1983)	18	13	Chemo	Acute
RTOG/EORTC-Acute (1984)	14	13	RT	Acute
RTOG/EORTC-Late (1984)	68	17	RT	Late
LENT/SOMA (1995)	140	13	RT	Late
CTC v2.0 (1998)	152	22	RT	Late
CTCAE v3.0 (2003)	260	22	All[a]	Acute
	370	All	All	Acute and late

WHO, World Health Organization; Chemo, chemotherapy; RT, radiation therapy.
[a] Limited pediatric and surgical criteria

specifying anatomic sites or other subclassifications, raises the number to 900 adverse effect criteria for grading. The need for a simplified summary toxicity methodology and a global adverse effect score, inclusive of multiple organ systems, has yet to be defined, and is essential for outcome reporting.

13.2
The Biologic Basis for Combining Acute and Late Criteria

The most prominent feature of CTCAE v3.0 is the merging of early and late effects criteria into a single uniform document and the development of criteria applicable to all modalities. The research support for the concept of a "biologic continuum" is based upon the original paradigm by Rubin and Casarett [10] in which the clinical radiation pathophysiologic course of events incorporating the a dynamic sequence of cellular events and tissue specific effects began at the moment of radiation exposure. The schema illustrated radiation effects, both the clinical and subclinical events, in each organ system, but noted that, depending on its cell population and tissue organization, would express radiation syndromes differently. The underlying pathophysiologic commonality was the obliteration of the normal tissues' fine microvasculature, whereas the time to clinical expression, the latent period, is related to stem cell depletion in either rapid or slow renewal systems, i.e., acute versus chronic or early versus late effects. This paradigm was the first formalism linking acute and late effects as both a pathophysiologic and a clinical biocontinuum. More recently, the molecular biologic events captured as a persistent cytokine cascade induced by radiation in a murine model has recapitulated the shape of the Rubin and Casarett tissue effect over time curves, adding further to their validity [11]. The arbitrary 90-day rule dividing 'early' and 'late' is no longer acceptable, since modalities overlap and are administered concurrently, and adjuvant chemotherapy is repeatedly cycled often for months and years. The use of a complex concurrent or hybrid sequential schedules undermines the usefulness of a simplistic temporally defined "early-late" construct. Moreover, there is growing recognition that surgery [12, 13] and chemotherapy [14], much like radiation, lead to molecular events resulting in a perpetual cytokine, chemokine cascade and surgery induces wound healing responses that result in inflammation, fibrogenesis, and neoangiogenesis, leading to epithelial regeneration. This multimodal molecular cascade leads to and supports the biologic continuum model (Fig. 13.1).

13.3
Validation, Standardization of Language, and Statistical Reporting

There is no universal agreement as to validation of content or construct to reliably quantify the injurious normal tissue effects following cancer treatment. A perceptive distinction of desirable properties of criteria for reporting and grading of toxicity

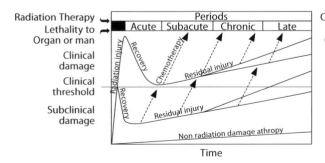
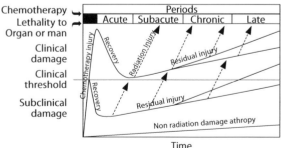

a   b

Fig. 13.1a,b. The clinicopathologic course of events following irradiation can be complicated by the addition of chemotherapy. Similarly, chemotherapy can result in parallel set of events. **a** Classically, when radiation therapy precedes chemotherapy, the introduction of the second mode can lead to expression of subclinical damage or, when injury is present, to death. **b** The same is true if chemotherapy precedes radiation therapy. (Reprinted from [15] with permission)

according to Bentzen are either explorative science-driven studies or clinical pragmatic patient-centered guidelines [16, 17]. Validation of toxicity criteria requires serial descriptions of adverse effects evolving over time (Fig. 13.2).

Using the terminology of numerical taxonomy requires defining the "operational taxonomic unit" (OTU) to decide on how to group toxicities of different organs into the same clusters or stages. One possibility is to utilize the impact on the host quality of life (QOL) scales, activities of daily living (ADL) or Karnofsky mobility ratings [18]. Ideally, any proposed system needs scientific study in clinical trials as to feasibility, reliability, specificity, responsiveness, as well as validity. Validity simply stated is whether a scale measures what is supposed to be measured. For routine reporting, peak prevalence of a specific morbidity as a function of time at a specific follow-up, i.e., 1–5 years or longer, is commonly noted, as is local regional cancer control and disease-free survival.

Longitudinal studies of the temporal evolution of late effects can provide either a cumulative incidence or, alternatively, Kaplan Meier [19] method for quantifying morbidity as a function of time. The search for early surrogate biomarkers and molecular biologic mechanisms that can predict late effects is clearly an important research direction [20].

Standardization of language requires use of the International Dictionary of Medical Terminology and commonly used disease codes, i.e., ICD 10 [21] and need to be synchronized with both CTC and LENT-SOMA diagnoses. Thus, the descriptors of adverse effects language can become more uniform and will reduce interinvestigator variability. The introduction of quality of life scales to represent the patients' viewpoint is an important aspect of grading adverse effects. Another important aspect is the need to integrate CTC and LENT-SOMA more fully. The LENT-SOMA is based on anatomic terms consisting of 15–20 major systems with approximately 50–60 subsites and is compatible, but not identical, with the terminology of the TNM system [22]. By contrast, the CTCAE v3.0 utilizes more physiologic and functional terms and clinical syndromes. There is as much concurrence and similarities as differences and a comparison of terms is presented in Table 13.2. The anatomical terminology reconciliation of the three systems is consistent with the International Anatomical Terminology (Terminologia Anatomica) approved in 1998 by the International Federation of the Association of Anatomists (Table 13.2) [23].

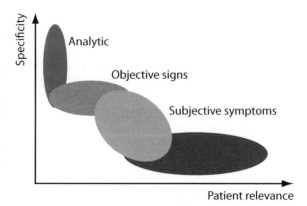

Fig. 13.2. Schematic representation of the trade-off between specificity and patient relevance of various dimensions of normal tissue effects. (Reprinted from [16] with permission)

Table 13.2. Anatomic-physiologic systems: hybrid nomenclature

Anatomic sites AJCC[a] TNM	Physiologic systems CTC v3.0[b]
Central nervous system	Neurology
(Neuroendocrine[b])	Endocrine
Ophthalmologic sites	Ocular/visual
Head and neck sites	Upper respiratory
Digestive system	Gastrointestinal
Major digestive glands	Hepato/biliary/pancreas
Thorax Breast	
Lung	
Pleura	Pulmonary
(Heart[b])	Cardiac, arrhythmia
(Vascular[b])	Vascular
Genitourinary sites	Renal/genitourinary Male sexual reproduction
Gynecologic sites	Female sexual reproduction
Musculoskeletal	Musculoskeletal
Skin	Dermatology, lymphatics
Lymphoid sites	Allergy, immunology
Bone marrow	Blood, bone marrow Hemorrhage, bleeding Infection, coagulation

[a] AJCC Cancer Staging Manual anatomic terms
[b] NCI CTC v3.0 are the basis for the physiologic terms. There are a number of unique terms in CTC v3.0 as syndromes, second malignancies, growth and development that do not fit into a hybrid anatomic/physiologic systems nomenclature

There is a large and growing literature assessing both the CTC systems and LENT-SOMA. Numerous clinical trials have been published often comparing these systems with other late toxicity grading criteria, particularly in Europe. The literature is equally divided between concordance and discordance in confirmation of their applicability. The majority of reports are retrospective and not prospectively designed to assess validation, especially for LENT-SOMA [24–32]. However, more recently, direct comparison has been made utilizing CTC v3.0 and LENT-SOMA. Furthermore, recent analysis from a validation perspective of clinical trials conducted at a variety of anatomic sites by RTOG confirms that LENT-SOMA is a superior instrument at capturing late effects. Utilizing a technique of linguistic analysis, there are 12 recurrent criteria that apply to grading most of the organ systems. The "shared" word descriptors for each grade, which can be identified in both LENT-SOMA and CTC v3.0, enable a "concise grading dictionary" of well-defined lexicons, capturing the essence of both systems. The SOMAtization of CTC v3.0 is shown in Table 13.3, which provides a more focused selection of criteria and should enable users to record toxicities more efficiently and accurately. The array of criteria relate to five categories: symptoms, physical findings, interventions to ameliorate, quality of life, or activities of daily living. Laboratory values and imaging studies are works in progress as regards correlations with gradations of toxicity and at this time should not override the other criteria when assigning grade.

13.4
Normal Tissue/Organ TNM Taxonomy for Adverse Effects of Cancer Treatment

13.4.1
TNM Language

There is a logic for adopting the TNM nomenclature for normal tissue/organ adverse effects following cancer treatment. The TNM language was introduced to allow for consistency in the classification and staging of cancer. The adoption by the American Joint Committee on Cancer (AJCC) and the International Union Against Cancer (UICC) 50 years ago has enabled oncologists worldwide to stratify patients, allow for multidisciplinary communication, better treatment decisions, and more accurate end results reporting. With a common language for cancer staging, cooperative oncology group protocols allowed for multimodal regimens to be designed and tested in clinical trials. The standardization of TNM staging nomenclature allows for evaluation and assessment of the literature. Therefore, a modification of this cancer nomenclature will be applied to normal tissue/organ toxicity.

Table 13.3. Somatization of CTCAE v3.0

	Mild Grade 1+	Moderate Grade 2+	Severe Grade 3+	Life Threatening Grade 4+
S	Asymptomatic Minimal symptoms	Symptomatic usually marked symptoms	Persistent symptoms Intensive symptoms	Refractory symptoms Symptoms unresponsive to medication
O	Transient signs Functionally intact	Intermittent signs Function altered	Symptoms apparent Function impaired	Advanced persistent signs Function collapsed
M	No interventions Occasional medication Occasional non-narcotic	Non-invasive intervention Continuous medication Regular non-narcotic	Interventional radiology Surgical correction Occasional narcotic	Radical life saving surgery Intensive care unit Parenteral narcotic
A	Normal laboratory values Borderline low, correctable BM cellularity < 25% decrease	Abnormal laboratory values, correctable BM cellularity > 25%–50%	Very abnormal lab Lab values not correctable BM cellularity > 50%, < 75%	Failing lab values Potentially lethal BM < 75%
ADL QOL	ADL regular KPS 80–100 Fully ambulatory	ADL Altered KP 60–75 Symptomatic, in bed < 50% day	ADL impaired KP 30–50 Symptomatic, in bed > 50%	ADL extremely poor KP 10–25 100% bedridden

13.4.2
General Rules

Philosophically, the TNM cancer classification is based on the premise that all malignant tumors progress from an early localized stage to a more disseminated later stage. The life cycle of all cancers shares in having a locus of origin in a normal tissue, which invades locally and advances to lymph nodes regionally and/or hematogenously to remote sites. In a parallel fashion, there is a similar life cycle for normal tissue reactions to multimodal cancer treatment. The normal tissues in which the cancer originated will be the target of surgery and radiation, as well as targeted chemotherapy. The neighboring normal tissue structures and sites in the region of lymph nodes are at risk and often have reactions to the aforementioned modalities, especially in concurrent regimens. Multiagent chemotherapy combinations are designed to diffuse the toxicity and can elicit systemic responses hematologically. Remote sites from the cancer can be affected, i.e., heart (Adriamycin), kidney (Cisplatinum), etc.

The practice of dividing cancer into "early versus late" was based on the progression from a localized stage to an advanced stage. In a parallel fashion, adverse effects also progress from "acute to late." Just as cancer is staged before treatment, the normal tissues – structure and function – need to be noted for baseline values and the presence of co-morbidities.

The proper staging of cancer applies to accurate recording of the status of host normal tissues and serves a number of related objectives, such as:
a) Selection of a corrective therapeutic intervention
b) Estimation of eventual prognosis
c) Assistance in evaluation of results of the intervention
d) Facilitates exchange of data amongst investigators
e) Of special importance to cancer control is establishing the therapeutic ratio

13.4.3
New Definitions of TNM Applied to Adverse Effects of Normal Tissue

The conceptual design of the $_N$TNM is similar to tumor spread into three compartments: primary tumor site, regional nodes, and systemic dissemination. The adverse effect of cancer treatment can be confined to the anatomic site of cancer origin or extend to involve other structures in the neighboring region or be a generalized or systemic toxic effect.

- $_NT$ = The normal Tissue, anatomic structure, organ in which the cancer arose and spreads initially.
- $_NN$ = Neighboring or surrounding normal tissues or organs, viscera that are not involved by the tumor but are in the regional nodal drainage zone.
- $_NM$ = SysteMic effects that are generalized and include hematologic, hepatic toxicity, weight loss.

Progression of the adverse effect can be designated numerically and becomes the operational taxonomy unit.

13.4.4
Assigning the Grade for Progression

The progression of a malignancy over time is designated by the assignment of numbers 1, 2, 3, 4 as subscripts to T and N, the primary tumor and nodal compartments, respectively. In an analogous fashion, the translation of late effects into a scale that allows for progression over time is important. The general guidelines are in the construction of criteria.

The operational taxonomic unit (OTU) is the grade assigned as applied according to criteria in CTCAE v3.0, LENT-SOMA or RTOG/EORTC scales which is 1+ mild, 2+ moderate, 3+ severe, or 4+ life threatening and will be determined by the degree of toxicity at each anatomic site or organ.

Grade 1+: Asymptomatic, signs are minimal and neither interfere with functional endpoints nor impede mobility. Most often, management is restrained, interventions and medication are not required.

Grade 2+: Symptomatic, moderate findings clinically or in the laboratory, that may alter functional endpoints without impact on QOL or ADL. Medications and non-surgical interventions can be used and be useful.

Grade 3+: Effects are indicative of severity of symptoms and signs, which persist over time. Disruption of mobility, working, and numerous functional endpoints. More serious interventions, such as hospitalization or surgery, are often indicated.

Grade 4+: Effects are potentially life threatening, catastrophic, disabling and result in loss of limb, bowel, or organ function.

Grade 5+: Fatal

Some more important principles established in CTC v3.0 are equally applicable to this proposed $_NT_NN_NM$ taxonomy:
- Acute and late effects merged in one system and applied with restrictive time applications.
- The system applies equally to all modalities.
- The duration or chronicity should be determined by serial longitudinal protocol studies.

When multiple normal structures are affected, each will be evaluated separately and be given a summary score. When multiple normal structures are involved and then compiled, a global toxicity score is derived.

13.4.5
Classification According to Evidence for Certainty of Grade

As in cancer classification, there are four types of classification depending on the diagnostic procedures and the relationship to the cancer treatment versus an intervention to manage the adverse effect. Clearly, the adverse normal tissue effect can be assessed before treatment, during, and immediately after multimodal treatment.
a) Clinical classification is based on physical examination, imaging, often with CT or MRI, endoscopy, and routine laboratory procedures. Minimally invasive procedures, such as needle aspiration, are useful and permissible. Most baseline values for vital normal tissues and assessments of acute and subacute reactions to multimodal treatment are in this category. $_{CN}$TNM
b) Pathologic classification requires an invasive procedure and, as in cancer staging an adverse chemoradiation effects, may require a surgical intervention and resection. Even surgical handling of vasculocompromised tissues may precipitate a necrotizing reaction as in exploring adherent bowel at laparotomy. Such invasive procedures are usually performed after multimodal cancer treatment to rule out recurrent cancers, which can masquerade as a late effect. PET or SPECT and MRI/MRS are valuable for establishing radiation sequelae as a confirmatory tissue diagnosis is critical [33, 34]. Biopsies, especially generous ones, may precipitate severe necrosis and need to be performed with caution.
c) Retreatment classification could apply to salvage cancer treatment, as well as management intervention to ameliorate the adverse effect. Either sophisticated imaging, such as PET/SPECT or MRI/MRS, can be of value to distinguish recurrence or persistence of cancer versus normal tissue necrosis [33, 34]. $_{RN}$TNM.
d) Autopsy classification: If death is attributed to an adverse effect, usually life threatening (4+) and fatal (5+), autopsy is mandatory to exclude incidental co-morbidities. According to Fajardo et al. [35], there are no pathognomic microscope features but certain constellations of radiation/chemotherapy stigmata; again, ruling out cancer recurrence is essential. $_{AN}$TNM
e) Prefixes and suffixes may be added in certain circumstances: An 'm' suffix indicates multiple structures, sites, and organs and may express the adverse effect, i.e., TN$_{(m)}$M. A 'y' prefix indicates an evaluation performed during or following initial multimodal therapy, i.e., $_{yp}$TNM.

13.4.6
Summary Toxicity Grade

Using the terminology of numerical taxonomy requires defining the "operational taxonomic unit" to decide how to group toxicities of different organs into the same clusters and stages [16].

The expansion of CTC v3.0 approaches a thousand descriptors, involving 15–20 major organ systems which, if divided into subsites (50–60), multiplies the elements and challenges investigators to offer a 'summary grade' for reporting outcomes. LENT-SOMA has a similar complex and detailed compilation of criteria. This has often been circumnavigated by utilizing the abbreviated late effects scales of the RTOG/EORTC cooperative groups. The operational taxonomic unit (OTU) is the number assigned to the grade of toxicity; however, the adverse late effect can vary over time. The biocontinuum of acute/late effects has been confirmed both in the laboratory measuring function in the clinic with physiologic testing. A rationale for selecting the OTU or summary grade of a specific organ system as a function of time in a longitudinal protocol (Fig. 13.3) would be to determine the area under the biocontinuum "effect-time curve" at specified time intervals, i.e., 2 years and 5 years [36].

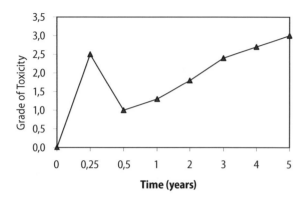

Fig. 13.3. Summary toxicity grade. The summary toxicity grade for a specific effect is a function of the grade of the effect over time. This can be recorded in three different parameters: (1) Maximal toxicity grade, (2) average grade over time, (3) area under the curve (grade x time)

13.4.7
Global Toxicity Score of Multiple Organs

Stage grouping is an important aspect of the staging of cancer and applies directly to adverse effects involving multiple sites. Because in cancer staging there are four Ts, three Ns and two Ms, there are 24 possible combinations. To recluster TN into the four stages I, II, III, IV would be a challenge when adverse effects are collated in multiple normal tissues.

The global toxicity score could be the compilation of the summary grades for each normal tissue assessed. With more than one structure in each of the defined zones, i.e., $_NT$ for site of cancer origin or

$_NN$ for site(s) of neighboring tissues

$_NM$ for systemic toxicities of system

The recommendation is to score each summary grade as noted and then add the subscripts. Thus, the global toxicity is the sum of subscripts and creation of stage grouping similar to staging cancers.

I = T1N1M1 or T2N1M0 or T3 N0M0
   = 1–3
II = T2N2M2 OR T3N1M0 OR T1N3M1
   = 4–6
III = T3N3M3 or T4N2M1 or T2N2+2M1
   = 7–9
IV = T4N4M4 or T3N2M1 or T2N2+2+3M1+2
   = 10–16, or
V = > 16

The complexity is in weighting the impact of numerous normal tissue/organ sites on quality of life and activities of daily living. Obviously, these recommendations and generalizations will need compilation of data from clinical trials before an accurate and meaningful global score can be arrived at.

13.4.8
Therapeutic Ratio Determination and Decision Making

In summary, a compelling reason for developing a parallel TNM system of staging adverse effects of normal tissue is to determine therapeutic ratios. An excellent illustration is when there is no survival advantage in competitive multimodal treatment programs, but one has less adverse effects. A recent report on advanced laryngeal cancers favored concurrent administration of cisplatinum and 5-fluorouracil followed by radiotherapy or surgery with the primary endpoint being laryngeal preservation, as well as local regional control, the latter being the same in the other arm [37]. Ideally, cure without complications is a function of cancer stage and the aggressiveness of the treatment. The classic figure of therapeutic ratio is a dose–response curve based on cancer control versus normal tissue injury with displacement to the left for cancer control and to the right for the normal tissue. The reality is the cancer control curves are displaced to the right as a function of cancer stage and cancer treatment becomes more aggressive leading to more complications, displacing normal tissue effects to the left. Thus, toxicity of treatment often increases as the cancer stage advances and the therapeutic window is often closed due to the crossover of curves.

References

1. American Cancer Society (1995) Cancer Facts and Figures 1995. Atlanta, American Cancer Society
2. Miller AB, Hoogstraten B, Staquet M et al (1981) Reporting results of cancer treatment. Cancer 47:207–214
3. Trotti A, Byhardt R, Stetz J et al (2000) Common toxicity criteria: Version 2.0. An improved reference for grading the acute effects of cancer treatment: Impact on radiotherapy. Int J Radiat Oncol Biol Phys 47:13–47
4. Cox JD, Stetz J, Pajak TF (1995) Toxicity criteria of the Radiation Therapy Oncology Group (RTOG) and the European Organization for Research and Treatment of Cancer (EORTC). Int J Radiat Oncol Biol Phys 31:1341–1346
5. Trotti A (2002) The evolution and application of toxicity criteria. Sem Radiat Oncol 12:1–3

6. Rubin P, Constine S, Fajardo L et al (1995) Overview of Late Effects of Normal Tissues (LENT) scoring system. Int J Radiat Oncol Biol Phys 31:1041–1042
7. Trotti A, Rubin P (2003) Introduction. Sem Radiat Oncol 13:175
8. Available at : http://ctep.info.nih.gov/CTC3/ctc.htm. Accessed April 1, 2003
9. Trotti A, Colevas DA, Setser A et al (2003) CTCAE v3.0: Development of a comprehensive grading system for the adverse effects of cancer treatment. Semin Radiat Oncol 13:176–181
10. Rubin P, Casarett GW (1968) Clinical Radiation Pathology. Philadelphia, PA, Saunders
11. Rubin P, Johnston CJ, Williams JP et al (1995) A perpetual cascade of cytokines postirradiation leads to pulmonary fibrosis. Int J Radiat Oncol Biol Phys 33:99–109
12. Fedyk ER, Jones D, Critchley HO et al (2001) Expression of stromal-derived factor-1 is decreased by IL-1 and TNF and in dermal wound healing. J Immunol 166:5749–5754
13. Mercado AM, Padgett DA, Sheridan JF et al (2002) Altered kinetics of IL-1, Il-1, and KGF-1 gene expression in early wounds of restrained mice. Brain Behav Immun 16:150–162
14. Petak I, Houghton JA (2001) Shared pathways: Death receptors and cytotoxic drugs in cancer therapy. Pathol Oncol Res 7:95–106
15. Rubin P (2001) Clinical Oncology. 8th ed. Philadelphia, PA, WB Saunders
16. Bentzen SM, Dörr W, Anscher MS et al (2003) Normal tissue effects: reporting and analysis. Semin Radiat Oncol 13:189–202
17. Trotti A, Bentzen MS (2004) The need for adverse effects reporting standards in oncologyclinical trials. J Clinc Oncol 22:19–22
18. Movsas B (2003) Quality of life in oncology trials: a clinical guide. Semin Radiat Oncol 13:189–202
19. Peters LJ, Withers HR, Brown BW (1995) Complicating issues in complication reporting. Int J Radiat Oncol Biol Phys 31:1349–1351
20. Williams J, Chen Y, Rubin P, Finkelstein J, Okunieff P (2003) The biological basis of a comprehensive grading system for the adverse effects of cancer treatment. In: JE Tepper (ed) The adverse effects of cancer treatment: metrics, management, and investigations. Semin Radiat Oncol 13:182–188
21. World Health Organization (1992) ICD 10: international statistical classification of diseases and related health problems, 10th ed. American Psychiatric Publishing
22. American Joint Committee on Cancer (AJCC) (2002) Cancer staging manual, 6th ed. Springer, Berlin Heidelberg New York
23. Federative Committee on Anatomical Terminology (FCAT) (1998) Terminologia anatomica: international anatomical terminology. Georg Thieme Verlag, Stuttgart
24. Davidson SE, Burns MP, Routledge JA et al (2003) Assessment of morbidity in carcinoma of the cervix: a comparison of the LENT SOMA scales and the Franco-Italian glossary. Radiother Oncol 69:195–200
25. Davidson SE, Burns MP, Routledge JA et al (2003) The impact of radiotherapy for carcinoma of the cervix on sexual function assessed using the LENT SOMA scales. Radiother Oncol 68:241–247
26. Routledge JA, Burns MP, Swindell R et al (2003) Evaluation of the LENT-SOMA scales for the prospective assessment of treatment morbidity in cervical carcinoma. Int J Radiat Oncol Biol Phys 56:502–510
27. Hoeller U, Tribius S, Kuhlmey A et al (2003) Increasing the rate of late toxicity by changing the score? A comparison of RTOG/EORTC and LENT/SOMA scores. Int J Radiat Oncol Biol Phys 55:1013–1018
28. Fehlauer F, Tribius S, Holler U et al (2003) Long-term radiation sequelae after breast-conserving therapy in women with early-stage breast cancer: an observational study using the LENT-SOMA scoring system. Int J Radiat Oncol Biol Phys 55:651–658
29. Denis F, Garaud P, Bardet E et al (2003) Late toxicity results of the GORTEC 94-01 randomized trial comparing radiotherapy with concomitant radiochemotherapy for advanced-stage oropharynx carcinoma: comparison of LENT/SOMA, RTOG/EORTC, and NCI-CTC scoring systems. Int J Radiat Oncol Biol Phys 55:93–98
30. Davidson SE, Burns M, Routledge J et al (2002) Short report: a morbidity scoring system for Clinical Oncology practice: questionnaires produced from the LENT SOMA scoring system. Clin Oncol (R Coll Radiol) 14:68–69
31. Anacak Y, Yalman D, Ozsaran Z et al (2001) Late radiation effects to the rectum and bladder in gynecologic cancer patients: the comparison of LENT/SOMA and RTOG/EORTC late-effects scoring systems. Int J Radiat Oncol Biol Phys 50:1107–1112
32. Tawfiq N, Lagarde P, Stockle E et al (2000) Conservative treatment of extremity soft tissue sarcomas. Functional evaluation using LENT-SOMA scales and Enneking scoring. Cancer Radiother 4:421–427 (French)
33. Bragg DG, Rubin P, Hricak H (2002) Oncologic imaging, 2nd ed. WB Saunders Company, Philadelphia
34. Husband JES, Reznek RH (1998) Imaging in oncology. ISIS Medical Media, Oxford
35. Fajardo LF, Berthrong M, Anderson RE (2001) Radiation pathology. Oxford University Press, USA, 2001
36. Movsas B, Scott C, Langer C et al (2005) Randomized trial of amifostine in locally advanced non-small-cell lung cancer patients receiving chemotherapy and hyperfractionated radiation: radiation therapy oncology group trial 98-01. J Clin Oncol. 23(10):2145-2154
37. Forestiere AA, Goepfert H, Maor M et al (2003) Concurrent chemotherapy and radiotherapy for organ preservation in advanced laryngeal cancer. N Engl J Med 349:2091–2098

Cancer Survivorship Research:
State of Knowledge, Challenges and Opportunities

Noreen M. Aziz

CONTENTS

14.1 Introduction *110*
14.2 Definitional Issues *110*
14.3 The Evolving Paradigm of Cancer Survivorship Research *111*
14.4 Long Term Cancer Survivors: Research Needs and Issues in a Growing Yet Understudied Portion of the Survivorship Continuum *112*
14.5 Cancer Survivors, Health Care Utilization, and Co-Morbid Conditions *113*
14.5.1 Metabolic Syndrome Associated Diseases – Obesity, Diabetes and Cardiovascular Disease *113*
14.5.2 Osteoporosis *114*
14.5.3 Decreased Functional Status *114*
14.5.5 Overview of Physiologic Sequelae of Cancer and its Treatment *115*
14.5.5.1 Physiologic Late Effects *115*
14.5.5.2 Second Cancers *117*
14.6 Follow-up Care for Late and Long-Term Effects *117*
14.7 Guidelines for Follow-Up Care – Issues and Strategies *119*
14.8 A Follow-Up Care Strategy Predicated on Research *122*
14.8.1 Follow-Up Care Research *122*
14.8.2 Development of Guidelines *123*
14.8.3 Implementation of a Guideline Based Follow-Up Care Strategy *123*
14.8.4 Caring for Long-Term Cancer Survivors *124*
14.9 Discussion *124*
14.10 Conclusion *127*
References *127*

N. M. Aziz, MD, PhD, MPh
Senior Program Director, Office of Cancer Survivorship Division of Cancer Control and Population, Sciences National Cancer Institute, Bethesda, MD 6130 Executive Boulevard, Bethesda, Maryland, 20892

Summary

With continued advances in strategies to detect cancer early and treat it effectively along with the aging of the population, the number of individuals living years beyond a cancer diagnosis can be expected to continue to increase. Most therapeutic modalities for cancer, while beneficial and often lifesaving against the diagnosed malignancy, are associated with a spectrum of late complications ranging from minor and treatable to serious or, occasionally, potentially lethal. Investigators conducting research among cancer survivors are reporting that long-term or late adverse outcomes of cancer and its treatment are more prevalent, serious, and persistent than expected in survivors of both pediatric and adult cancer. However, these adverse sequelae remain poorly documented and understood, especially among those diagnosed as adults. These findings underscore the need for continued cancer survivorship research.

This paper examines:
- Definitional issues relevant to cancer survivorship
- The evolving paradigm of cancer survivorship research
- Research needs and issues of particular relevance to long-term cancer survivors
- Cancer survivorship as a scientific research area, with an overview of physiologic/medical sequelae of cancer diagnosis and treatment, and
- Follow up care and surveillance of cancer survivors,

Both length and quality of survival are important end points for the large and ever-growing community of cancer survivors. Interventions—therapeutic and lifestyle—may carry the potential to treat or ameliorate adverse outcomes, and must be developed, examined and disseminated if found effective.

14.1 Introduction

With continued advances in strategies to detect cancer early and treat it effectively along with the aging of the population, the number of individuals living years beyond a cancer diagnosis can be expected to continue to increase [1, 2, 3, 4]. In the absence of other competing causes of death, 66% of adults diagnosed with cancer today can expect to be alive in 5 years [5]. Relative 5 year survival rates for those diagnosed as children (age <19 y) are even higher, with almost 79% of childhood cancer survivors estimated to be alive at 5 years, and 75% at 10 years [6, 7, 8, 9]. Medical and socio-cultural factors such as psychosocial and behavioral interventions, active screening behaviors, and healthier lifestyles may also play an integral role in the length and quality of that survival [10, 11].

Most therapeutic modalities for cancer are associated with a spectrum of late complications ranging from minor and treatable to serious or, occasionally, potentially lethal [3, 4, 12]. Thus, there is today a greater recognition of symptoms that persist after the completion of treatment and also those that arise years after primary therapy. Both acute organ toxicities such as radiation pneumonitis and chronic toxicities such as congestive cardiac failure, neurocognitive deficits, infertility and second malignancies are being described as the price of cure or prolonged survival. The study of late effects, originally within the realm of pediatric cancer, is now germane to cancer survivors at all ages because concerns may continue to surface throughout the life cycle. These concerns underscore the need to follow-up, monitor and screen survivors of cancer for toxicities such as those mentioned and also to develop and provide effective interventions that carry the potential to prevent or ameliorate adverse outcomes [3, 4].

The goal of survivorship research is to focus on the *health and life* of a person with a history of cancer *beyond* the acute diagnosis and treatment phase. Survivorship research seeks to examine the causes of, and to prevent and control the adverse effects associated with, cancer and its treatment, and to optimize the physiologic, psychosocial, and functional outcomes for cancer survivors and their families. A hallmark of survivorship research is its emphasis on understanding the integration/interaction of multi-disciplinary domains.

This paper will: present definitional issues relevant to cancer survivorship; describe the evolving paradigm of cancer survivorship research; explore research needs of particular relevance to long-term cancer survivors; examine cancer survivorship as a scientific research area; provide a brief overview of medical sequelae of cancer diagnosis and treatment; assess the impact of these adverse sequelae on post-treatment follow-up care; and articulate gaps in knowledge and emerging research priorities in cancer survivorship research.

14.2 Definitional Issues

Fitzhugh Mullan, a physician diagnosed with and treated for cancer himself, first described cancer survivorship as a concept [13]. Definitional issues for cancer survivorship encompass two related aspects: *1) What is cancer survivorship?* Mullan described the survivorship experience as similar to the seasons of the year. He recognized three seasons or phases of survival: *acute* (extending from diagnosis to the completion of initial treatment, encompassing issues dominated by treatment and its side effects), *extended* (beginning with the completion of initial treatment for the primary disease, remission of disease, or both; dominated by watchful waiting, regular follow-up examinations and, perhaps, intermittent therapy) and *permanent* survival (not a single moment; evolves from extended disease-free survival when the likelihood of recurrence is sufficiently low). An understanding of these phases of survival is important for facilitating an optimal transition into and management of survivorship; and *2) What is cancer survivorship research?* Cancer survivorship research seeks to identify, examine, prevent, and control adverse cancer diagnosis and treatment-related outcomes (such as late effects of treatment, second cancers and quality of life); provide a knowledge base regarding optimal follow-up care and surveillance of cancer survivors; and optimize health after cancer treatment.

Other important definitions include those for *long-term cancer survivorship* and *late versus long-term effects of cancer treatment*. Generally, *long-term cancer survivors* are defined as those individuals who are 5 or more years beyond the diagnosis of their primary disease and embody the concept of permanent survival described by Mullan. *Late effects* refer specifically to unrecognized toxicities that are absent or sub-clinical at the end of therapy and become manifest later with the unmasking of hitherto unseen injury due to any of the following factors: developmental processes; the failure of compensatory mechanisms with the passage of time; or, organ senescence. *Long-term effects* refer to any side effects or complications of treatment for which a cancer patient must compensate; also known as persistent effects, they begin during treatment and continue beyond the end of treatment. Late effects, in contrast, appear months to years after the completion of treatment. Some researchers classify cognitive problems, fatigue, lymphedema and peripheral neuropathy as long-term effects while others classify them as late effects [14, 15, 16, 17].

14.3 The Evolving Paradigm of Cancer Survivorship Research

Consistent with the shift in our perceptions of cancer as a chronic disease, new perspectives, and an emerging body of scientific knowledge must now be incorporated into Mullan's original description of the survivorship experience [2, 3, 4, 13]. Mullan's comparison of cancer survivorship with "seasons of the year" had implied that the availability and widespread use of curative and effective treatments would lead to a low likelihood of recurrence and longer survival times. However, the potential impact of late and long-term adverse physiologic and psychosocial effects of treatment was not described. In addition, further advances in survivorship research over the past few years have necessitated the incorporation of other emerging concepts into the evolving paradigm of cancer survivorship research [2, 3, 4]. These include: the impact of comorbidities on a survivor's health status and their possible interaction with risk for or severity of late effects; the key role of lifestyle factors and health promotion in ameliorating adverse treatment and disease-related consequences; the effect of cancer on the family; and the need for incorporating a developmental and life-stage perspective in order to facilitate optimally a cancer patient's journey into the survivorship phase. A developmental/life-stage perspective is particularly important as it carries the potential to affect and modify treatment decisions, the intensity of post-treatment follow-up care, the risk and severity of adverse sequelae of treatment, and the need for or use of technologies such as sperm banking (depending on the survivor's age at diagnosis and treatment) [2, 3, 4]. Data on late effects from studies conducted largely in childhood cancer survivors [18] have paved the way for and provided an implied "paradigm" for cancer survivorship research among adult survivors. Whether there is a consistent childhood cancer survivorship model requires examination. If this is so, we must explore whether and to what extent it holds true for adult and elderly survivors; the distribution, determinants and health implications of late effects among adults; and similarities or differences in outcomes of cancer and its treatment between pediatric and adult cancer survivors.

It is of critical importance that we design and conduct cancer survivorship research with methodologic rigor. Confounders, effect modifiers, mediators, and moderators need to be assessed. Measurement issues are challenging and multifaceted. Not only must late and long-term medical effects be measured, attention also needs to be directed to the careful assessment of concurrent co-morbid conditions. The impact of late or long-term effects on the timing and severity of co-morbid conditions, and vice versa, needs to be examined rigorously. Health related quality of life needs to be assessed in conjunction with late effects and co-morbid conditions. Thus, these measurement issues are complex and encompass at least 3 inter-related aspects of cancer survivorship. All this needs to be carried out with an overall research/theoretical model that is capable of explaining the results and inferences observed [2, 3, 4].

Major portions of the published literature on cancer survivorship are descriptive (hypothesis generating) in nature. Survivorship research studies should now move towards analytic (hypothesis testing) study designs, clinical trials and interventions. Creative hybrid designs such as nested case-control or case-cohort studies are of great value in yielding quantitative data. Triangulation of methodologies, utilizing a combination of qualitative and quantitative approaches, are also immensely useful. There is a need for exploring models for interventions that are effective and can be disseminated into the community, and a need for education both for the provider and the survivor. Educational needs include the development of guidelines for optimal post-treatment follow-up care and monitoring of pediatric and adult cancer survivors, and the prevention, early detection, or management of late and long-term effects of cancer treatment. These guidelines must be evidence-based, and evaluated for effectiveness and impact.

The constantly evolving effect of a philosophical shift in cancer treatment from a primarily seek-and-destroy mindset toward one reflecting the importance of both curing the disease and controlling its attendant adverse sequelae significantly affects the cancer survivorship research paradigm of the new millennium. Cancer treatments today are increasingly used in the context of the survivor's life, striving toward minimal toxicity yet optimal effectiveness and with a recognition of the importance of interdisciplinary care and management. This philosophy must be communicated to researchers and care providers across diverse settings to promote its incorporation into the design of the next generation of cancer survivorship investigations [2, 3, 4].

Thus, our new, dynamic, and evolving paradigm of cancer survivorship research can be summarized as one that:
- Seeks to identify, examine, prevent and control adverse sequelae of cancer and its treatment
- Manages, treats and prevents comorbidities
- Incorporates health promotion and lifestyle interventions to optimize health after cancer treatment
- Defines optimal follow-up care and surveillance strategies and guidelines for all survivors
- Pays special attention to disparities in survivorship outcomes by age, income, ethnicity, geography or cancer site, and
- Explores the impact of the survivorship experience on the family (and vice versa).

This paradigm looks *beyond* treatment, representing a shift away from a medical deficit-dysfunction model, and towards a multi/inter disciplinary focus. Cancer survivorship research studies now rarely examine late effects in isolation, and are beginning to, and will continue to, incorporate the full domains of cancer survivorship research (physiologic, psychosocial, economic) in their conceptual models and research designs. There is a desire and a need to elucidate the underlying mechanisms, biology and bio-behavioral basis of sequelae, and the competing causes of morbidity and mortality. As such, cancer survivorship research today reflects the incredible successes in cancer treatment and early detection that have enabled the continued growth in numbers of cancer survivors and their expectation to lead rich and fruitful lives [2, 3, 4].

14.4
Long Term Cancer Survivors: Research Needs and Issues in a Growing Yet Understudied Portion of the Survivorship Continuum

Despite the increasing number of cancer survivors living 5 years or more after a cancer diagnosis, a review of the literature indicates that most of what we know about cancer survivorship today focuses largely on the period between diagnosis and 2 years after treatment (the early survivorship phase). However, most late effects of cancer treatment have much longer latency periods, [3, 9, 10, 11, 12, 13, 19] and tend to occur during the extended survivorship years. Thus, while cancer survivors are living longer, we have limited knowledge and many questions about the health status, functioning, and quality of life for most of those who have been post-treatment for long periods of time: What are the most common late effects of treatment? Who is at risk and can they be protected? Can treatment-related injury to normal tissue be prevented or reversed? What proportion of survivors will experience recurrent or second malignancies? Who should be following these survivors for disease recurrence? What constitutes "optimal surveillance" and what is the cost of such follow-up care? Do medical, psychosocial, or behavioral interventions reduce morbidity in these populations? These questions, especially among those diagnosed with cancer as adults, underscore the need for continued research in this ever-growing portion of the cancer survivorship spectrum [9, 10, 11, 13, 21].

To date, the prevalence, incidence, relative risk, and genetic basis of late and long-term effects of cancer and its treatment among survivors diagnosed at least 5 years ago remains to be elucidated for the majority of cancer sites. Among adults, the largest body of knowledge comes from breast cancer survivors. Highly prevalent primary cancer sites such as colorectal, gynecologic, head and neck, prostate and lung continue to be understudied with respect to medical outcomes such as: cardiotoxicity, [20, 21] neurocognitive problems, [22, 23, 24, 25] premature menopause, [26] sexual impairment, [27, 28] infertility, [29, 30] chronic fatigue, [31, 32] pain syndromes, and second malignancies [33].

There is growing appreciation of the role that socio-cultural and behavioral factors play in patient outcomes, decision-making, adherence to treatments, and willingness to adopt appropriate surveillance and health maintenance behaviors post-treatment. Psychosocial or behavioral interventions carry the potential to improve the health-related quality of life, functioning and even medical status of cancer survivors and their family members [34, 35]. While we know that human behavior can have a profound impact on how cancer is managed and may also affect disease-free or overall survival, we are not currently using this information in the systematic delivery of care. We also know little about the best delivery of interventions, and we continue to need more data regarding psychosocial issues such as poor quality of life, fear of recurrence, poor self-esteem, anxiety and depression, job lock or loss, employment and insurance discrimination, body-image disturbances, relationship difficulties, and financial hardship [36, 37, 38, 39, 40].

Survivorship outcomes among medically underserved and ethno-culturally diverse cancer survivor populations, and family members or care-givers, represent another under-studied area [24, 41, 42]. Although more than 62% of cancer survivors are age 65 and older, and the median age at diagnosis is 67–68 years, only a fraction of research studies have examined the effect of cancer and its treatment on older individuals. This major segment of the cancer survivor population also tends to be affected by co-morbid health conditions which may interact with the cancer treatment itself, and may modulate the risk for, or severity of, persistent or late effects of cancer therapy [43].

Finally, while high quality follow-up care is a necessary fact of life for all cancer survivors, both for the prevention or early detection of physiological and psychosocial sequelae, and for the timely introduction of optimal treatment strategies to prevent or control late effects, to-date, there is no standardized model of service delivery applied consistently across cancer centers and post-treatment follow-up care programs. Nor has an attempt been made to examine the quality, content, and optimal frequency of follow-up care of cancer survivors delivered in the community setting by oncologists or by primary care providers [44].

Areas of emphasis and potential research questions in long-term cancer survivorship research are presented in Table 14.4.

14.5
Cancer Survivors, Health Care Utilization, and Co-Morbid Conditions

Cancer survivors are high healthcare utilizers affecting distinct healthcare domains owing to therapeutic exposures, genetic predisposition and/or lifestyle risk factors [3, 4, 10, 45, 46, 47]. While the threat of progressive or recurrent disease is at the forefront of health concerns for a cancer survivor, increased morbidity and decreased functional status and disability that result from cancer, its treatment or health-related sequelae also are significant concerns. The impact of chronic co-morbid conditions on cancer and its treatment is heightened more so among those diagnosed as adults and those who are elderly at the time of diagnosis.

Presented below is a brief overview of some factors potentiating the risk for chronic co-morbid conditions among cancer survivors. A brief discussion of the major co-morbid illnesses observed among survivors is also presented.

14.5.1
Metabolic Syndrome Associated Diseases – Obesity, Diabetes and Cardiovascular Disease

Obesity is a well-established risk factor for cancers of the breast (post-menopausal), colon, kidney (renal cell), esophagus (adenocarcinoma), and endometrium, thus a large proportion of cancer patients tend to be overweight or obese at the time of diagnosis [48, 49] Additional weight gain also can occur during or after active cancer treatment, an occurrence that has been frequently documented among individuals with breast cancer, but recently has been reported among testicular and gastrointestinal cancer patients, as well [50, 51]. Given data that obesity is associated with cancer recurrence in both breast and prostate cancer, and reduced QOL among survivors, there is compelling evidence to support weight control efforts in this population [52, 14, 15]. Gradual weight loss also has proven benefits in controlling hypertension, hyperinsulinemia, pain, dyslipidemia, and improving levels of physical functioning – conditions that reportedly are significant problems in the survivor population [53, 14, 15, 21]

Obesity is a common manifestation of several metabolic disorders that are frequently observed among cancer survivors. These disorders are grouped under the umbrella term, "the metabolic syndrome", and also include diabetes and cardiovascular disease (CVD). Insulin-resistance is the underlying event associated with the metabolic syndrome and co-occurs with hyperinsulinemia and/or diabetes [54, 55, 56]. Diabetes may play an especially significant role in the increased number of non-cancer related deaths among survivors, however, its role in progressive cancer is still speculative [3, 4].

Older breast cancer patients may derive a cardioprotective benefit from their diagnosis and/or associated treatments (most likely due to tamoxifen) [57]. Reports indicate that CVD is a major health issue among survivors, evidenced by mortality data which show that half of non-cancer related deaths are attributed to CVD [10]. Risk is especially high among men with prostate cancer who receive hormone ablation therapy, as well as patients who receive adriamycin, and radiation treatment to fields surrounding the heart [58].

14.5.2
Osteoporosis

Osteoporosis and osteopenia are prevalent health conditions in the general population, especially among women. Despite epidemiologic findings that increased bone density and low fracture risk are associated with an increased risk for breast cancer [59, 60, 61, 62] clinical studies suggest that osteoporosis remains an important health concern among survivors [63, 64] Approximately 80% of older breast cancer patients have t-scores less than –1 and thus have clinically confirmed osteopenia at the time of their initial appointment. Other cancer populations, such as premenopausal breast and prostate cancer patients may possess good skeletal integrity at the onset of their disease, but are at risk of developing osteopenia which may ensue with treatment-induced ovarian failure or androgen ablation [10].

14.5.3
Decreased Functional Status

Previous studies indicate that functional status is lowest immediately after treatment and tends to improve over time; however, the presence of pain and co-occurring diseases may affect this relationship [65]. In the older cancer survivor, regardless of duration following diagnosis, the presence of comorbidity, rather than the history of cancer per se correlates with impaired functional status [66]. Cancer survivors demonstrate almost a two-fold increase in having at least one functional limitation, and, in the presence of another co-morbid condition, the odds ratio increases to 5.06 (95% CI 4.47-5.72) [67]. These findings have been confirmed by other studies in diverse populations of cancer survivors [68, 69, 70]

Survivors of childhood cancer may experience an increased risk for functional limitations in physical performance and participation in activities of daily living. Compared with siblings, survivors are more likely to report performance limitations, restricted participation in personal care skills, problems with routine activities, and an adverse impact on the ability to attend work or school [71]. They also suffer from significantly elevated rates of *chronic* health conditions. Approximately 62.3% of 10,397 survivors in a recent study had at least one chronic, while 27.5% had a severe or life-threatening, condition. The cumulative incidence of a chronic health condition was 73.4%, and for a severe, disabling, or life-threatening condition was 42.4%, even as late as 30 years after diagnosis [72].

Among survivors diagnosed as adults, a seminal study utilizing the Nurses Health Study Cohort was the first to report that breast cancer results in persistent declines in multiple dimensions of functional health status, and that socially isolated and younger women are an especially vulnerable group. These prospective data suggest that previous studies reporting no difference in physical function among breast carcinoma cases compared with disease free women underestimated the deleterious effect of the disease on function [73] After adjustment for age, baseline functional health status, and multiple covariates, women who developed incident breast carcinoma were more likely to have experienced reduced physical function, role function, vitality, and social function and increased bodily pain compared with women who remained free of breast carcinoma. The risk of decline was attenuated with increasing time since diagnosis. Risk of decline in physical function was evident across all stages of breast carcinoma, even after adjustment for women undergoing treatment for persistent or recurrent disease. Compared with women < or = 40 years without breast cancer, women with breast cancer experienced significant functional declines. Young (age < or = 40) women who developed breast cancer experienced the largest relative declines in HRQoL (as compared with middle-aged and elderly women) in multiple domains including physical roles, bodily pain, social functioning and mental health [74]. Among socially isolated women, role function, vitality, and physical function were significantly lower compared to the most socially integrated women. Prediagnosis level of social integration was also shown to be an important factor in future HRQoL among breast cancer survivors [75].

14.5.5
Overview of Physiologic Sequelae of Cancer and its Treatment

14.5.5.1
Physiologic Late Effects

Late and long-term effects can be classified further as: *(a) system specific* (such as damage, failure or premature aging of organs, immunosuppression or compromised immune systems, and endocrine damage); *(b) second malignant neoplasms* (such as an increased risk of a certain cancer associated with the primary cancer and a second cancer associated with cytotoxic or radiological cancer therapies); *(c) functional changes* (such as lymphedema, incontinence, pain syndromes, neuropathies and fatigue); *(d) cosmetic changes* (such as amputations, ostomies and skin and hair alterations); and *(e) associated comorbidities* (such as osteoporosis, arthritis, scleroderma and hypertension) [1, 2, 3, 4]. The risk of a recurrence of the primary malignancy also must be kept in mind.

Generalizations: Certain types of late effects can be anticipated from exposure to specific therapies, age of the survivor at the time of treatment, combinations of treatment modalities and dosage administered [20]. Susceptibility differs for children and adults. Generally, chemotherapy results in acute toxicities that can persist, whereas radiation therapy leads to sequelae that are not immediately apparent. Combinations of chemotherapy and radiation therapy are more often associated with late effects. Toxicities related to chemotherapy, especially those of an acute but possibly persistent nature, can be related to proliferation kinetics of individual cell populations because these drugs are usually cell-cycle dependent. Organs or tissues most susceptible have high cell proliferation rates and include the skin, bone marrow, gastrointestinal mucosa, liver and testes. The least susceptible organs and tissues replicate very slowly or not at all and include muscle cells, neurons and connective tissue. However, neural damage may be caused by commonly used chemotherapeutic drugs such as methotrexate, vinca alkaloids and cytosine arabinoside; bone injury may be caused by methotrexate; and cardiac sequelae can occur after treatment with adriamycin. Injuries in tissues or organs with low repair potential may be permanent or long lasting. Risk of late death from causes other than recurrence is greatest among survivors treated with a combination of chemotherapy and radiotherapy [1, 2, 3, 4]. The *most frequently observed medical sequelae* include endocrine complications, growth hormone deficiency, primary hypothyroidism, primary ovarian failure, cardiac dysfunction, neurocognitive deficits and second cancers. Risk factors for late effects may act independently or synergistically.

Issues unique to certain cancer sites: The examination of late effects for childhood cancers such as leukemia, Hodgkin's lymphoma and brain tumors have provided the foundation for this area of research. A body of knowledge on late effects of radiation and chemotherapy is also now appearing for adult cancer sites such as *breast cancer*. For example, neurocognitive deficits that may develop after chemotherapy for breast cancer are an example of a late effect that was initially observed among survivors of childhood cancer receiving cranial irradiation, chemotherapy or both [3, 9, 10, 11, 33, 34]. We now have preliminary support for the hypothesis that the epsilon 4 allele of APOE may be a potential genetic marker for increased vulnerability to chemotherapy-induced cognitive decline [76]. Late effects of bone marrow transplantation have been studied for both adult and childhood cancer survivors as have sequelae associated with particular chemotherapeutic regimens for Hodgkin's disease and breast cancer [3, 20, 35, 36]. The side effects of radiotherapy, both alone and with chemotherapy, have been reported fairly comprehensively for childhood cancer sites associated with good survival rates. Most cancer treatment regimens consist of chemotherapy in conjunction with surgery or radiation, and multidrug chemotherapeutic regimens are the rule rather the exception. As such, the risk of late effects must always be considered in light of all other treatment modalities to which the patient has been exposed.

Issues unique to specific therapeutic exposures: The use of *anthracyclines* for cancer treatment is associated with cardiotoxic effects among survivors of both childhood and adult cancer. The result is cardiomyopathy and potentially irreversible congestive heart failure. Anthracycline-induced cardiotoxicity is characterized by reduced left ventricular wall thickness and mass, indicating decreased cardiac muscle and depressed left ventricular contractility. Risk factors include high cumulative doses, high dose intensity, and radiotherapy. Among survivors of breast cancer, *Herceptin* and *radiotherapy* have both been shown to exert cardiotoxic effects. Cardiomyopathy disease progression can be delayed in adults by using angiotensin-converting enzyme inhibitors such as enalapril. Studies in long-term survivors of pediatric cancer has shown that enalapril has significant benefits in preventing cardiac functional deterioration on a short-term basis, but this is not sustained. Dexrazoxane may significantly reduce cardiotoxicity associated with anthracyclines in adult patients, and is possibly efficacious among children and adolescents as well. Significantly fewer dexrazoxane-treated patients (21%) had elevated serum cardiac troponin (a biomarker of acute myocardial injury) levels than patients treated with chemotherapy alone (50%; P <.001). Dexrazoxane has been shown to have no effect on the event-free survival rate at 2.5 years, emphasizing that it does not detrimentally affect the efficacy of anthracycline therapy [77, 78, 79, 80]. However, its long-term impact on the risk for second cancers remains to be elucidated. In terms of health-related quality of life, important differences have been reported between breast cancer survivors treated with chemotherapy compared to local therapy alone, suggesting that long-term QOL may vary depending on the type of treatment and diagnosis [81].

Special considerations when primary diagnosis and treatment occurs in childhood: Cancer therapy during childhood may interfere with physical and musculoskeletal development, [82, 83, 84, 85, 86] neurocognitive and intellectual growth, [87, 88] and pubertal development [89]. These effects may be most notable during the adolescent growth spurt. Prevention of second cancers is also a key issue [11, 13].

Premature menopause is a frequent and significant after effect of cancer treatment. It has now been shown that childhood cancer survivors who retain ovarian function after completing cancer treatment are at increased risk of developing premature menopause (cessation of menses before age 40 years). Risk factors for such nonsurgical premature menopause include attained age, exposure to increasing doses of radiation to the ovaries, increasing alkylating agent score (based on number of alkylating agents and cumulative dose), and a diagnosis of Hodgkin lymphoma. Those treated with alkylating agents plus abdominopelvic radiation are at particularly high risk (cumulative incidence approaching 30%) [90] Defined as the loss of ovarian function within 5 yr of diagnosis, acute ovarian failure is known to develop in a subset of survivors of pediatric and adolescent cancers. Risk factors for acute ovarian failure include: older age at diagnosis, Hodgkin's lymphoma, and, abdominal or pelvic radiotherapy in doses of at least 1000 cGy. Increasing doses of ovarian irradiation, exposure to procarbazine, and exposure to cyclophosphamide at ages 13–20 yr have also been reported as independent risk factors [91].

Special considerations when primary diagnosis and treatment occurs during adulthood: Some late effects of chemotherapy may assume special importance depending on the adult patient's age at the time of diagnosis and treatment [3]. Diagnosis and treatment during the young adult or early reproductive years may call for a special cognizance of the importance of maintaining reproductive function and the prevention of second cancers [92].

Cancer patients diagnosed and treated in their 30s and 40s may need specific attention for premature menopause; issues relating to sexuality and intimacy; use of estrogen replacement therapy; prevention of neurocognitive, cardiac and other sequelae of chemotherapy; and prevention of coronary artery disease and osteoporosis [3, 11, 20]. Sexual dysfunction may persist after breast cancer treatment and may include vaginal discomfort, hot flashes and alterations in bioavailable testosterone, luteinizing hormone and sex hormone binding globulin [93]. Menopausal symptoms such as hot flashes, vaginal dryness and stress urinary incontinence are very common in breast cancer survivors and cannot be managed with standard estrogen replacement therapy in these patients. The normal life expectancy of survivors of early-stage cancers during these years of life underscores the need to address their long-term health and quality-of-life issues [3, 9, 10].

Although *older patients (aged 65 years or more)* bear a disproportionate burden of cancer, advancing age is also associated with increased vulnerability to other age-related health problems, any of which could affect treatment choice, prognosis and survival. The combination of late effects of cancer or its treatment and age-related health problems and co-morbidities add to the vulnerability of older survivors. In one study, older or long-term survivors who had chemotherapy and survivors with more types of treatment reported significantly more symptoms both during treatment and currently. Women and African Americans appear to be at special risk for more symptoms and greater functional difficulty. Pain was the most commonly reported symptom, with 21% attributing it to cancer [94]. Hence, cancer treatment decisions may have to consider preexisting or concurrent health problems (comorbidities). Measures that can help to evaluate comorbidities reliably in older cancer patients are warranted. Little information is available on how comorbid age-related conditions influence treatment decisions and the subsequent course of cancer or the comorbid condition. It is also not known how already compromised older cancer patients tolerate the stress of cancer and its treatment and how comorbid conditions are managed in light of the cancer diagnosis [52].

14.5.5.2
Second Cancers

Second cancers may account for a substantial number of new cancers. A second primary cancer is associated with the primary malignancy or with certain cancer therapies (e.g., breast cancer after Hodgkin's disease or ovarian cancer after primary breast cancer) [1, 2, 3, 4]. Within 20 years, survivors of childhood cancer have an 8–10% risk of developing a second cancer [1, 2, 3, 4]. This can be attributed to the mutagenic risk of both radiotherapy and chemotherapy, which is further compounded in patients with genetic predispositions to malignancy. The risk of a second cancer induced by cytotoxic agents is related to the cumulative dose of drug or radiotherapy [1, 2, 3, 4]. The risk of malignancy with normal aging may be a result of cumulative cellular mutations. The interaction of the normal aging process and exposure to mutagenic cytotoxic therapies may result in an increased risk of second malignancy, particularly after radiotherapy and treatment with alkylating agents and podophyllotoxins. Commonly cited second cancers include leukemia after alkylating agents and podophyllotoxins; solid tumors, including breast, bone and thyroid cancer in radiation fields; and bladder cancer after cyclophosphamide. Second cancers may also occur in the same organ site (e.g., breast, colorectal); thus there is a clear need for continued surveillance [3, 9, 10, 73].

14.6
Follow-up Care for Late and Long-Term Effects

Optimal follow-up of survivors includes both an ongoing monitoring and assessment of persistent and late effects of cancer treatment, and the successful introduction of appropriate interventions to ameliorate these sequelae [44]. The achievement of this goal is challenging, and inherent in that challenge is the recognition of the importance of preventing premature mortality from the disease and / or its treatment, and the prevention or early detection of both the physiologic and psychologic sources of morbidity. The prevention of late-effects, second cancers, and recurrences of the primary disease requires watchful follow up and optimal utilization of early detection screening techniques. Physical symptom management is as important in survivorship as it is during treatment and effective symptom management during treatment may prevent or lessen lasting effects [1, 2, 3, 4, 44, 95].

Regular monitoring of health status post cancer treatment is recommended since this should 1) permit the timely diagnosis and treatment of long-term complications of cancer treatment; 2) enable timely diagnosis and treatment of recurrent cancer; 3) facilitate screening for, and early detection of, a second cancer; 4) allow the detection, and referral for management, of co-morbid conditions; and 5) provide the opportunity to institute preventive strategies such as diet modification, tobacco cessation and other life style changes [1, 2, 3, 4, 44, 104, 105]

Quality continuing care for cancer survivors spans a broad spectrum of medical domains ranging from surveillance to genetic susceptibility [1, 2, 3, 4, 44, 104, 105, 96]. Health promotion, since it addresses modifiable factors, is a key concern of survivors once acute management of their disease is complete. Increasingly, cancer survivors are looking to their oncology care providers for counsel and guidance with respect to lifestyle change that will improve their prospects of a healthier life, and possibly a longer one as well. While complete data regarding lifestyle change among cancer survivors have yet to be determined, and there remains an unmet need for behavioral interventions with proven efficacy in various cancer populations, [97] the oncologist can nonetheless make use of extant data to inform practice and also should be attentive to new developments in the field.

Follow-up care and monitoring for late effects is usually done more systematically and rigorously for survivors of childhood cancer while they continue to be part of the program or clinic where they were treated. The monitoring of adult cancer sites for the development of late effects, particularly outside the oncology practice, is neither thorough nor systematic. It is important that survivors of both adult and childhood cancers be monitored for the late and long-term effects or treatment discussed in preceding sections, at regular intervals.

While it is now recognized that cancer survivors may experience various late physical and psychological sequelae of treatment, and that many health care providers may be unaware of the adverse outcomes, [98] until recently, there were no clearly defined, easily accessible risk-based guidelines for cancer survivor follow-up care. Such clinical practice guidelines can serve as a guide for doctors, outline appropriate methods of treatment and care, address specific clinical situations (disease-oriented) or use of approved medical products, procedures, or tests (modality-oriented). In response to this growing mandate, the Children's Oncology Group has developed and published its guidelines for long-term follow-up for Survivors of Childhood, Adolescent, and Young Adult Cancers [99]. These risk-based, exposure-related clinical practice guidelines are intended to promote earlier detection of and intervention for complications that may potentially arise as a result of treatment for pediatric malignancies, and are both evidence-based (utilizing established associations between therapeutic exposures and late effects to identify high-risk categories) and grounded in the collective clinical experience of experts (matching the magnitude of risk with the intensity of screening recommendations). Importantly, they are intended for use beginning 2 or more years following the completion of cancer therapy, and are not intended to provide guidance for follow-up of the survivor's primary disease.

Of great significance to survivors of adult cancer, using the best available evidence, ASCO's expert panels have also identified and developed practice recommendations for post-treatment follow-up of specific cancer sites (breast and colorectal; source: www.asco.org). In addition, ASCO has also created an expert panel tasked with the development of follow-up care guidelines geared towards the prevention or early detection of late effects among survivors diagnosed and treated as adults.

It is critical, if we are to develop effective research priorities and recommendations for clinical care, education, and policy related to care for survivors of cancer, that we note two key points: (a) the population of cancer survivors consists of individuals with varying needs and issues - those cured of their disease and no longer undergoing active treatment, as well as patients with recurrences or resistant disease requiring ongoing treatment; and (b) regardless of disease status, any survivor may experience lasting adverse effects of treatment [100].

Survivors of cancer have significantly poorer health outcomes on multiple burden-of-illness measures than do people without a history of cancer, and these health decrements may occur or continue many years after diagnosis [1, 2, 3, 4, 44] Co morbid conditions are another major issue for many diagnosed with cancer, yet little is known about the quality of the non-cancer-related care receive by these survivors [101]. Compared with matched controls with no history of cancer, it has been reported that it is more likely that survivors would not receive recommended care across a broad range of chronic medical conditions (e.g., angina, congestive heart failure, and diabetes) [5]. Quality-of-life issues in long-term survivors of cancer differ from the problems they face at the time of diagnosis and treatment [102, 103]. Thus, interventions with the potential to treat or ameliorate these many and varied late and chronic effects of cancer and its treatment must be developed, evaluated for efficacy, and disseminated.

The larger scientific community has begun to champion the need for cancer survivorship research, and to call for solutions that will lead to both increased length and quality of life for all cancer survivors. This demand is reflected in the language of several Institute of Medicine (IOM) and President's Cancer Panel reports, Progress Review Group (PRG) documents, and National Cancer Institute priorities. The IOM Report on cancer survivors diagnosed as adults articulates key areas for research and care delivery, especially with respect to the development of a formal care plan for survivors that integrates, within one document, key treatment relevant variables, exposures, late effect risks, and management/follow-up care needs [104]. The recent IOM report on childhood survivorship cites the need to create and evaluate standards and alternative models of care delivery, including collaborative practices between pediatric oncologists and primary care physicians as well as hospital-based long- term follow-up clinics [105]. Another IOM Report, *Ensuring Quality Cancer Care*, recognized that attributes of high quality care could be linked to optimal outcomes such as enhanced length and quality of survival, and that continued medical follow-up of survivors should include basic standards of care that address the specific needs of long-term survivors.

Survivors of cancer who have completed initial therapy generally require significant amounts of follow-up care during the first two years of diagnosis. The frequency and intensity of monitoring diminishes each year thereafter, a dramatic decrease occurring 2–5 years post-treatment. Conversely, the risk of late effects and the impact of long-term effects increases with time. This progressive fall-off in cancer and non-cancer related medical visits may reflect either a failure of the medical system to convey the risk for adverse treatment-related sequelae, or a manifestation of system driven barriers (unequal access, disparities in receipt of quality care). Patient driven factors (fear of recurrence or of findings) are also critical. Not all survivors may be aware of the late effects they may be at risk for. Thus treating physicians and institutions must provide survivors with a discharge summary detailing key treatment/exposure and baseline health information that may be relevant if or when late effects become manifest. They must also develop a tailored follow-up care plan that reflects elevations in risk due to previous therapeutic exposures.

To facilitate optimal follow-up during the post-treatment phase, the patient's age at diagnosis, side effects of treatment reported or observed during treatment, calculated cumulative doses of drugs or radiation, and an overview of late effects most likely for a given patient given the treatment history, should be summarized and kept on file. A copy of this summary should be provided to the patient, or parent of a child who has undergone treatment for cancer. The importance of conveying this detailed treatment history to primary care providers should be clearly communicated, especially if follow-up will occur in the primary/family care setting. Finally, screening tests that may help detect subclinical effects that could become clinically relevant in the future should be listed.

The majority of cancer survivors return to their primary care providers for medical follow-up once treatment ends, many of whom may be unaware of the additional health risks of cancer treatment. Provider education and training is thus necessary. Extant published international long term follow-up care guidelines provide a logical basis for informed practice, but are not truly evidence based and must be updated regularly and communicated optimally to providers and survivors to be truly effective and useful [106, 107].

Due to the potential health vulnerability and complexity of medical needs, attention may shift away from important health problems not related to cancer, or, surveillance may become over vigilant. The lack of evidence base that can help tailor optimal care strategies needs to be addressed. The relative roles of primary care providers and specialists in the care of cancer survivors are not clear. Developing and testing interventions that examine outcomes among groups of survivors managed under different follow-up care settings is a critical need. We must add to the growing knowledge base of cancer survivorship and to facilitate the development of evidence based follow-up care and surveillance strategies in this health vulnerable group of individuals.

It is imperative that we achieve an evidence based understanding of the frequency, content, setting and experiences of follow-up care received by the broader population of cancer survivors in order to develop standards for such care with a view towards preventing, detecting early, or ameliorating the adverse outcomes [1, 2, 3, 4, 44]. Findings from methodologically rigorous studies will improve our understanding of the nature and extent of the burden of illness carried by cancer survivors, yield key information regarding follow-up care, and facilitate future efforts focusing on the development of standards or best practices for such care, especially when notable health disparities might exist.

Potential late effects of cancer and its treatment are summarized by organ system and by exposure to chemotherapy, radiation, or surgery, in Table 14.1. Suggested follow-up care and monitoring strategies and guidelines for the prevention, early detection, or optimal management of late effects, are presented in Table 14.2.

14.7
Guidelines for Follow-Up Care – Issues and Strategies

The long-term and late effects of combined modality cancer treatment present important issues we must address through clinical research [108]. While awareness of late effects after cancer and agreement that they need to be prevented, managed or treated is increasing, many questions remain. We still do

Table 14.1. Possible Late Effects of Radiotherapy & Chemotherapy

Organ System	Late Effect/Sequelae of Radiotherapy	Late Effect/Sequelae of Chemotherapy	Chemotherapeutic drugs responsible
Bone and Soft Tissues	Short stature; atrophy, fibrosis, osteonecrosis	Avascular necrosis	Steroids
Cardiovascular	Pericardial effusion; pericarditis; CAD	Cardiomyopathy; CCF	Anthracylines Cyclophosphamide
Pulmonary	Pulmonary Fibrosis; Dec. Lung Volumes	Pulmonary fibrosis Interstitial pneumonitis	Bleomycin, BCNU Methotrexate, Anthracyclines
CNS	Neuropsychological Deficits, Structural Changes, Haemorrhage	Neuropsychological Deficits, Structural changes; Hemiplegia; seizure	Methotrexate
Peripheral Nervous System	-	Peripheral neuropathy; hearing loss	Platinum analogues, Vinca alkaloids
Hematological	Cytopenia, myelodysplasia	Myelodyplastic syndromes	Alkylating agents
Renal	Dec. creatinine clearance; Hypertension	Dec creatinine clearance; Inc. creatinine; Renal F Delayed Renal F	Platininum analogues Methotrexate Nitrosoureas
Genitourinary	Bladder fibrosis, contractures	Bladder fibrosis; Hemorrhagic cystitis	Cyclophosphamide
Gastrointestinal	Malabsorption; stricture; Abnormal LFT	Abnormal LFT; Hepatic fibrosis; cirrhosis	Methotrexate, BCNU
Pituitary	Growth hormone deficiency; pituitary deficiency	-	-
Thyroid	Hypothyroidism; nodules	-	-
Gonadal	Men: risk of sterility, Leydig cell dysfunction. Women: ovarian failure, early menopause	Men: sterility Women: sterility, prem menopause	Alkylating agents Procarbazine
Dental/oral health	Poor enamel & root formation; dry mouth	Tooth decay	Multiple
Opthalmological	Cataracts; retinopathy	Cataracts	Steroids

Table 14.2. Follow-up Care and Surveillance for Late Effects

Follow-up Visit	Content of Clinic Visit	Suggested Evaluative Procedures and Ancillary Actions
Chemotherapy/ Radiotherapy Treatment Completion	1. Review Complete Treatment History 2. Calculate cumulative dosages of drugs 3. Document Regimen(s) administered and Radiation ports, dosage, machine 4. Document patient age at diagn/Trt 5. Assess side effects during treatment 6. Identify likely late effects 7. Perform Baseline "grading" of late effects (CTCAEv.3.0, Garre, SPOG, others)	Develop late Effect Risk profile Summarize all information in previous column Provide copy to patient (or parent if minor child) Instruct that this summary should be provided to primary care or other health care providers Keep copy of summary in patient chart
General Measures at every visit	Detailed history Complete Physical exam Review systems Meds, maint., prophylactic antibiotics Education: GPA, school performance Employment history Menstrual status/cycle Libido, sexual activity Pregnancy & outcome	Evaluate symptomatology, patient reports of issues Review any intercurrent illnesses Evaluate for disease recurrence, second neoplasms Systematic Evaluation of long term(persistent) and late effects (See Specific Measures) Grade long term & late effects: Garre or SPOG criteria and note changes CBC; Urinalysis; Other tests depending upon exposure History and late effect risk profile

...continued Table 14.2.

Follow-up Visit	Content of Clinic Visit	Suggested Evaluative Procedures and Ancillary Actions
Specific Measures to evaluate late effects Relevance differs by: 1. Age at diagnosis/ Treatment 2. Specific drugs, regimens 3. Combinations of Treatment modalities 4. Dosages administered 5. Expected Toxicities (based on mech of action of cytotoxic drugs (cell cycle dependent; proliferation kinetics). 6. Exceptions occur to the theoretical assumption that least susceptible organs/tissues are those that replicate slowly or not at all (Platinum analogues, methotrexate, anthracyclines). 7. Combinations of radiation/chemotherapy more often associated with late effects.	Growth: Includes issues such as short stature, scoliosis, hypoplasia	Monitor growth (growth curve); sitting height, parental heights, nutritional status/diet, evaluate scoliosis, bone age, growth hormone assays, thyroid function, endocrinologist consult; orthopaedic consult (if appropriate)
	Cardiac	EKG, Echo, afterload reduction, cardiologist consult Counsel against isometric exercises if high risk, advise OB/Gyn risk of cardiac failure in pregnancy
	Neurocognitive	History and Exam Communicate: School, Family, Special education Compensatory Remediation Techniques Neuropsych consult; CT or MRI; CSF; basic myelin protein Written instructions, appointment cards
	Neuropathy	History/Exam: Neurolog exam, sensory ch hands/feet, paresthesias, bladder, gait, vision, muscle strength Neurologist consult
	Gonadal toxicity	History for primary vs. secondary dysfunction, gonadal function (menstrual cycle, pubertal development/delay, libido); hormone therapy; interventions (bromocriptine) Premature menopause: hormone replacement unless contraindicated; DXA scans for osteoporosis; calcium Endocrinologist consult Reproductive Technologies
	Pulmonary	Chest X-ray; Pulmonary function tests; Pulmonologist consultation
	Urinary	Urinalysis; BUN/Creatinine; Urologist if hematuria
	Thyroid	Annual TSH; thyroid hormone repl; Endocrinologist
	Weight History	Evaluate Dietary intake (Food diary)/Physical Activity Nutritionist and/or Endocrinologist consult
	Lymphedema	History/ Exam: swelling, Sensations of heaviness/fullness
	Fatigue	Rule out hypothyroidism; anemia, cardiac/pulm sequelae, Evaluate sleep habits; Evaluate physical fitness and activity levels Regular physical activity unless contra-indicated
	Surgical Toxicity	Antibiotic prophylaxis (splenectomy)
	Gastrointestinal/Hepatic	Liver function, hepatitis screen, Gastro-enterologist consult
Screening for Second Malignant Neoplasms	Screening guidelines differ by age Oncologist Consult	Follow guidelines for age appropriate cancer screening (mammogram, pap smear, FOBT/ Flex Sig) Mammog at age 30 if hx of mantle radiation for hodgkins Screen for associated cancers in HNPCC family syndrome Screen for ovarian cancer if hx of Breast ca and BRCAI II.
Assess/Manage Co-morbidities	Osteoporosis; Heart Disease; Arthritis, etc.	History/Exam; Be Cognizant of risk; Appropriate Consult;

not know what the overall burden of late effects is for survivors. The interaction between aging and late adverse effects is another key area that needs examination. What is becoming clear is that the severity of late effects shows a considerable interpatient variability.

To-date, it is impossible to predict at the start of cancer treatment the extent to which an individual patient will develop late or long-term effects od cancer treatment. The assessment of genetic susceptibility to the effects of radiation or chemotherapy may in the future enable us to understand better the nature of this interpatient variability [109, 110, 111].

While the primary goal of cancer treatment is cure or at least long-lasting palliation, at its most basic level, the principal aims of long-term follow-up after cancer care are prevention, early diagnosis and management of morbidity related to cancer or its therapies. Ongoing research on long-term effects after cancer will hopefully enable the establishment of an optimal balance between the laudable goal of cure or long-term palliation and the risk of inevitable long-term sequelae.

Cost-effective guidelines need to be established that take into account the different cancer types, an individual patient's risk of long-term toxicity, and the knowledge that the absolute number of long-term survivors with severe problems appears to be relatively low. A major issue that impacts guideline development is that fact that many severe late effects become clinically recognizable after latency periods of 10 years or more. Thus, a critical challenge that must be overcome relates to the involvement of primary care practitioners in the long-term follow-up of cancer survivors.

At present, there are no general guidelines that address the followup of long-term cancer survivors. While we continue to see valuable results concerning long-term morbidity after cancer, follow-up guidelines are by and large directed towards the detection of relapse and improvement of cancer-free survival. Some international guidelines have begun to recommend cooperation between the primary care sector and oncologists in order to strengthen the quality of long-term rehabilitation for cancer survivors. They have also suggested "national follow-up centers" for long-term cancer survivors that will not only conduct research relevant to the diagnosis, prevention and treatment of long-term side-effects, but will also provide medical care to those experiencing adverse effects and develop relevant guidelines for follow-up of cancer survivors [112].

14.8
A Follow-Up Care Strategy Predicated on Research

The plausible follow-up care strategy for long-term cancer survivors can be developed incrementally based on Four steps:

14.8.1
Follow-Up Care Research

Includes describing by person, place and time various types of late or long-term effects, and assessing their incidence and prevalence, relationship with the previous cancer, and pathophysiology. It needs to be kept in mind that not all morbidity observed among cancer survivors is related to the cancer experience, and that it may well be a consequence of aging or an unhealthy life style. Thus, comparison with age- and gender- matched normal population cohorts is key.

Patient- and treatment-related heterogeneity is a major challenge in follow-up care research: A multitude of factors contribute to morbidity in cancer survivors. These include environmental factors, life style (smoking, nutrition, physical activity) and patient-related variables such as age, gender and hormones [1, 2, 3, 4, 113, 114]. In addition, the variability of tumour sites, variable treatments and variations in responsiveness to treatment increase the complexity of follow-up care research in cancer survivors.

Methodologically, research strategies relevant to follow-up care may include retrospective cross-sectional studies (cost-effective) or, ideally, be based on longitudinal investigations with repeated examinations of cohorts of interest. Cross-sectional studies among cancer survivors generally require the establishment of an age- and gender-matched control group in order to identify the cancer-specific late toxicity. This type of study design is used for generating new hypotheses, whereas longitudinal studies enable a causal evaluation of long-term trends regarding the development of late effects. Models for longitudinal studies utilized for answering such questions include repeated surveys among clearly defined large populations and allow a comparison of cancer survivors' incidence and prevalence of late effects with a cancer-free population [115, 116]. In one study, authors compared health problems in cancer patients with those of the cancerfree individuals based on data as registered in the Cancer

Registry of Norway. However, they found that information on treatment data and extent of the disease tended to be incomplete [117, 118].

Thus, registry-based studies need to be supplemented by more detailed clinical studies evaluating the impact of overall treatment, pretreatment co-morbidity and major post-treatment health events. Questionnaire-based surveys among cancer survivors from population-based studies should be combined with clinical examinations which (if HIPAA regulations are complied with) also provide the possibility of collect biological material for the assessment of genetic and biochemical profiles that will allow an increased understanding of pathophysiological pathways.

A third strategy enabling follow-up care research might be include the use of data from large phase III clinical trials. In such studies, a large cohort is usually identified and characterized by relatively similar pre-treatment eligibility criteria and standardised treatment modalities. Another benefit of this approach is that cancer survivors from large phase III trials are regularly monitored resulting in longitudinal data which could be helpful in the understanding of intermediate steps leading to possible late effects.

14.8.2
Development of Guidelines

Guidelines should be created in an attempt to translate evidence from research into practice. Such guidelines should address the *frequency* of follow-up visits, *content of care* (examinations, tests) provided at each visit, and determine the *level/intensity* of health care to be provided based on a survivors' risk profile. Follow-up care guidelines should also outline the essential features of a written (a) Treatment Summary, and (b) Survivorship Care Plan to be given to a survivor at 2 time points: (i) the end of acute cancer treatment; and (ii) the end of specialist oncological care.

A Survivorship Care Plan should contain information regarding a survivor's treatment, complications observed or expected, the overall risk of adverse late or long-term effects, and steps/strategies whereby these adverse sequelae can be prevented, detected early, managed, or treated.

Clinical guidelines are systematically developed statements to assist specialists, general practitioners and patients to make decisions regarding appropriate health care for cancer survivors [119]. Their intent should be to decrease adverse health effects related to cancer and to enhance health and quality of life. Evidence-based guidelines are based on linkage between the therapeutic exposure and observed late effects and their risk factors. They also include screening recommendations. Guidelines for post-treatment follow-up care of long-term cancer survivors should, at the very least, include recommendations for a) monitoring of health status; b) surveillance relevant to the prevention or early detection of recurrence; c) early detection of late or long-term effects; d) treatment of late or long-term effects; e) detection of and referrals for the management of co-morbidities; and f) recommendations regarding life style adjustments. It should also be noted that since cancer therapies have evolved over time in relation to the type of cancer, and also in response to a patient's age, follow-up care guidelines must incorporate the impact of these key issues/sources of variability [120].

14.8.3
Implementation of a Guideline Based Follow-Up Care Strategy

Communication with the community health care professionals and ensuring their appropriate education and training regarding the late or long-term effects of cancer and its treatment and the unique health needs of cancer survivors are essential requirements for translating guidelines into clinical practice. Thus, an implementation strategy for guidelines should take into consideration these issues, along with an assessment of resources available.

General practitioners' adherence to guidelines is critical when translating recommendations into clinical practice [121]. Many clinicians may be unwilling to change their routine, or may have concerns about patient (survivor) or peer resistance. Implementation of guidelines and their adoption implies a permanent change in the manner "work" (follow-up care) was done previously. One way of changing is to follow the plan-do-study-act-cycle (PDSA-cycle) (www.ihi.org) which tests a change in the real work-setting by 1) planning the change, 2) trying it, 3) observing the results and 4) acting on what is learned. After testing the change in a small scale and refining the change through several PDSA cycles, the change is ready for use on a broader scale. Thus, the development and implementation of guidelines might begin with one malignancy and then be gradually expanded to other cancer types.

14.8.4
Caring for Long-Term Cancer Survivors:

It has been said that care across the cancer continuum implies longitudinal care from diagnosis until death, regardless of the patient's age [121]. The first phase of caring for long-term survivors includes treatment planning which takes into consideration, for individual patients, the balance between responsiveness to treatment and the risk of acute and late complications. Once long-term survival is achieved maintenance of "health that is as good as possible" and prevention of cancer- and treatment- related morbidity is the intention of the second phase. In this phase care should include physical, psychological, and social services. It should also include information and education of survivors" regarding their "new reality" predicated on a changed or evolving risk profile due to the cancer or its treatment and strategies that might reduce these challenges to health. Models of care which take into account the optimal frequency and intensity of follow-up for individual survivors need to be developed and tested [2, 4, 44, 95, 122].

High- and low- risk cancer survivors should be identified according their potential of developing late effects. Low-risk cancer survivors may be referred to the primary care specialist for further follow-up care, whereas high-risk cancer survivors may need follow-up at late effect clinics. The referral to primary care requires an ongoing guidance from the original oncologist with respect to the monitoring and management of late effects within a shared care model [44, 123]. Contact between the primary care and the late effects clinic should be encouraged, perhaps on an annual basis either by phone, mail or e-mail.

The complexity of long-term or late effects makes the care for cancer survivors time-consuming, which may make it difficult to integrate follow-up care into a busy primary care practice. The development of a Survivorship Care Plan may be the first step to facilitate the incorporation of long-term care for cancer survivors by primary care practitioners (community care). This document should include a brief summary of salient facts regarding the original treatment of the cancer itself, and be an evolving document in which details of further treatments or maintenance therapies should also be recorded. Further, it should include a presentation of possible late effects, and procedures to monitor and prevent them.

It should always be kept in mind that cancer survivors may have reservations about the benefits of follow-up care. Barriers precluding adherence to follow-up care may include negative emotions associated with reminders of the cancer experience at each follow-up visit. Even though it has been postulated that the experience of cancer increases the willingness to make life style changes, the persistence of such psychological attitude over years remains unclear.

14.9
Discussion

Cancer survivorship research continues to provide us with a growing body of evidence regarding the unique and uncharted consequences of cancer and its treatment among those diagnosed with this disease. It is becoming an acknowledged fact that most cancer treatment options available and in use today will affect the future health and life of those diagnosed with this disease. Adverse cancer treatment-related sequelae thus carry the potential to contribute to the ongoing burden of illness, health care costs, and decreased length and quality of survival [2, 44].

Given the current gaps in our knowledge, it is especially critical that we expand and accelerate our potential to address the impact of survival from cancer in particular with respect to:

- *Research questions addressing specific gaps in our knowledge*: such as the incidence of and risk factors for late and long-term effects of cancer and its treatment, role of socio-cultural and behavioral factors in modulating treatment outcomes, impact of survivorship on health care utilization, role of co-morbidity in outcomes, appropriate follow up care and surveillance for survivors, and the effect on families of living with a cancer history in a loved one; and,
- *Research among understudied survivor groups*: such as those treated for colorectal, gynecologic, or hematologic malignancies, and those belonging to underserved populations (e.g. adult, elderly, rural, low education/income, and diverse racial and ethnic populations) [2].

The goal of cancer survivorship research is to examine questions and develop interventions or strategies that will lead to a decrease in physiologic and psychologic morbidity and mortality associated with post-treatment survival from cancer. While there is a critical need for additional data on adult cancer survivors, innovative studies addressing gaps in research among survivors of childhood cancer, especially those who are 5 years or more beyond diagnosis, are also important. The next generation of survivorship studies will need to use appropriately valid and reliable measures of both physiologic and psychosocial variables. Furthermore, as the number of new therapies for cancer with as yet undocumented sequelae continue to increase, we will need research models and trained researchers poised to explore and address these [1, 2, 4].

Cancer survivorship research domains are presented in Table 14.3 and examples of research questions of particular relevance to long-term cancer survivorship are summarized in Table 14.4.

Table 14.3. Domains of Cancer Survivorship Research

Survivorship Research Domain	Definition and Potential Research Foci
Descriptive and analytic research	- Documenting for diverse cancer sites the prevalence and incidence of physiologic and psychosocial late effects, second cancers and their associated risk factors. Physiologic outcomes of interest include late and long-term medical effects such as cardiac or endocrine dysfunction, premature menopause and the effect of other comorbidities on these adverse outcomes Psychosocial outcomes of interest include the longitudinal evaluation of survivors' quality of life, coping and resilience, spiritual growth
Intervention research	- Examining strategies that can prevent or diminish adverse physiologic or psychosocial sequelae of cancer survivorship - Elucidating the impact of specific interventions (psychosocial, behavioral or medical) on subsequent health outcomes or health practices
Examination of survivorship sequelae for understudied cancer sites	- Examining the physiologic, psychosocial, and economic outcomes among survivors of colorectal, head and neck, hematologic, lung, or other understudied sites
Follow-up care and surveillance	- Examining the impact of high quality follow-up care on early detection or prevention of late effects - Elucidating whether the timely introduction of optimal treatment strategies can prevent or control late effects - Evaluating the effectiveness of follow-up care clinics / programs in preventing or ameliorating long-term effects of cancer and its treatment - Evaluating alternative models of follow-up care for cancer survivors - Developing a consistent, standardized model of service delivery for cancer related follow-up care across cancer centers and community oncology practices - Assessing the optimal quality, content, frequency, setting, and provider of follow-up care for survivors
Economic sequelae	- Examining the economic effect of cancer for the survivor and family and the health and quality-of-life outcomes resulting from diverse patterns of care and service delivery settings
Health disparities	- Elucidating similarities and differences in the survivorship experience across diverse ethnic groups - Examining the potential role of ethnicity in influencing the quality and length of survival from cancer.
Family and caregiver issues	- Exploring the impact of cancer diagnosis in a loved one on the family and vice versa
Instrument development	- Developing Instruments capable of collecting valid data on survivorship outcomes and developed specifically for survivors beyond the acute cancer treatment period - Developing / testing tools to evaluate long-term survival outcomes; and those that (i) Are sensitive to change, (ii) Include domains of relevance to long-term survivorship, (iii) Will permit comparison of survivors to groups of individuals without a cancer history and/or with other chronic diseases over time. - Identifying criteria or cut-off scores for qualifying a change in function as clinically significant (for example improvement or impairment)

Table 14.4. Areas of Research Emphasis in Long-term Cancer Survivorship Research* (examples only)

Area of Research Emphasis	Potential Research Questions
A) Research related to specific survivor groups (i) Those treated for previously understudied cancer sites (e.g. colorectal, gynecologic, hematologic, head and neck, lung), (ii) Those belonging to understudied or underserved populations (adult, elderly, rural, low education/income, and diverse racial and ethnic populations).	- What are the late or persistent effects of cancer and its treatment in older adult (65 years or older) long term cancer survivors? - What is the health status, functioning, and quality of life of long term cancer survivors belonging to diverse cancer sites? - Which are the most common chronic and late effects among survivors across diverse cancer sites and which may be unique to subsets of different cancer survivor groups? - What are the characteristics of long-term survivors from rural communities and those from low income and educational backgrounds? - What are the similarities and differences in the survivorship experience among underserved cancer survivors and Caucasian survivors?
B) Research addressing specific gaps in our knowledge: In particular as related to: (i) Physiologic late or long-term effects	(i) Physiologic late or long-term effects - Who is at risk for late and long-term effects and can they be protected? Are there specific, modifiable risk factors (other than exposure to treatment) for the development of late effects? - Which sub-groups of adult cancer survivors are at elevated risk for declines in functional status? - What are the most common late physiological sequelae of cancer and its treatment among adults, and their effect on physical and psychosocial health? - To what extent does cancer treatment accelerate age-related changes? - Do co-morbidities affect risk for, development of, severity and timing of late effects of cancer treatment among adult cancer survivors? - What proportion of survivors will experience recurrent or second malignancies?
(ii) Psychosocial effects	(ii) Psychosocial effects - What are the psychosocial and behavioral consequences of late and or long-term physiological sequelae for survivors' health and well-being? - Which factors promote resilience and optimal well-being in survivors and their families?
(iii) Interventions	(iii) Interventions - Which interventions (medical, educational, psychosocial or behavioral) are most effective in preventing or controlling late or long term physiologic or psychosocial effects? When in the course of illness or recovery should they be delivered and by whom? - Can interventions delivered years after treatment control, reduce, or treat chronic or late cancer related morbidity?
(iv) Health Behaviors	(iv) Health Behaviors - Does regular physical activity after cancer (or avoidance of weight gain after hormonally dependent cancers) increase length and quality of survival? - Does having a cancer history alter cancer risk behaviors among long term survivors (e.g., smoking, alcohol consumption, sunscreen use)?
(v) Impact of Cancer on Family members	(v) Impact of Cancer on Family members: - What long-term impact does cancer have on the functioning and well-being of family members of survivors?
(vi) Post Treatment Follow-up Care, Surveillance, and Health Care Utilization	(vi) Post Treatment Follow-up Care, Surveillance, and Health Care Utilization - Who is currently following cancer survivors for disease recurrence, and cancer treatment-related late and long-term effects? - What is the optimal frequency, content, and setting of post-treatment medical surveillance of cancer survivors, especially for those who are adults, and by whom should it be delivered? - How does cancer history affect subsequent health care utilization, both cancer-related and that associated with co-morbidities?
C) Research that takes advantage of existing survivor cohorts or study populations	- Comparison of survivors' functioning over time and/or with other non-cancer populations (e.g., cohort or nested case-control studies).

14.10 Conclusion

As the number of survivors with long overall or disease-free survival periods increase, long-term health issues are fast emerging as a public health concern. Research on the chronic or delayed complications of cancer and its treatment or care is needed, and will: inform our understanding of the biology of the disease; lead to the design of novel, less toxic treatments; test the effectiveness of interventions – medical, pharmacologic, and behavioral – to reduce adverse physiological and quality of life outcomes; guide follow-up care practices; and inform patient and provider treatment-related decision making.

To-date, few studies have examined and compared survivor outcomes pre-and post diagnosis. Inferences such as those from the Nurse Health Study need to be examined among other populations of survivors (e.g. colorectal, prostate, gynecologic, etc). Future studies also need to be cognizant of and utilize a life stage framework. The special vulnerability among older or long-term survivors is an important issue researchers and clinicians need to address. To improve overall health and to prevent or control long term or late effects, many cancer survivors may need to initiate and maintain diet, exercise and other lifestyle changes soon after diagnosis, and strategies that will facilitate these changes need to be tested and disseminated.

Not only do the late and long-term consequences of cancer and its treatment occupy a central core of importance in and of themselves, they also can influence infrastructure systems such as databases, follow-up requirements in clinical practice settings or clinical trials, new therapeutic approaches, surveillance recommendations, and the cancer research agenda itself.

References

1. Aziz NM. Cancer survivorship research: challenge and opportunity. J Nutr, 132(11): 3494S-503S; 2002.
2. Aziz NM, Rowland JH. Trends and Advances in Cancer Survivorship Research: Challenge and Opportunity. Seminars in Radiation Oncology, 2003; 13(3): 248-66.
3. Aziz NM. Long-Term Survivorship: Late Effects. Chapter 71. Principles and Practice of Palliative Care and Supportive Oncology. Ann M Berger, Russell K. Portenoy, and David E. Weissman, eds. Philadelphia, PA. Lippincott Williams & Wilkins, 2006. 3rd Edition. Pages 787-804.
4. Aziz NM. Late Effects of Cancer Treatments: Surgery, Radiation Therapy, Chemotherapy. Chapter 101. Oncology: An Evidence-Based Approach. AE Chang, PA Ganz, DF Hayes, T Kinsella, HI Pass, JH Schiller, R Stone, and V Strecher, eds. New York, NY. Springer-Verlag, 2006. Pages 1768-1790.
5. American Cancer Society (2007). Cancer Facts and Figures, 2003, American Cancer Society Atlanta, GA.
6. Ries, L.A.G. Smith, M. A. Gurney, J. G. Linet, M. Taura, J. Young, J. L. Bunin, G. R. eds. Cancer incidence and survival among children and adolescents: United States SEER program 1975-1995. NIH Pub. No. 99-4649 National Cancer Institute, SEER Program Bethesda, MD.
7. Chu, K. C., Tarone, R. E. & Kessler, L. G. (1996) Recent trends in U.S. breast cancer incidence, survival, and mortality rates. J. Natl. Cancer Inst. 88:1571-1579.
8. McKean, R. C., Feigelson, H. S. & Ross, R. K. (2000) Declining cancer rates in the 1990s. J. Clin. Oncol. 18:2258-2268.
9. Aziz, N. M. (2002) Long-term survivorship: late effects. Berger, A. M. Portenoy, R. K. Weissman, D. E. eds. Principles and Practice of Palliative Care and Supportive Oncology 2nd ed. 2002:1019-1033 Lippincott Williams & Wilkins Philadelphia, PA.
10. Demark-Wahnefried W, Aziz NM, Rowland JH, Pinto BM. Riding the Crest of the Teachable Moment: Promoting Long-Term Health after the Diagnosis of Cancer. J Clin Oncol, 2005; 23:5814-5830.
11. Demark-Wahnefried, W., Peterson, B. & McBride, C. (2000) Current health behaviors and readiness to pursue life-style changes among men and women diagnosed with early stage prostate and breast carcinomas. Cancer 88:674-684.
12. Ganz PA. Late effects of cancer and its treatment. Semin Oncol Nurs. 2001 Nov;17(4):241-8.
13. Mullan, F. (1985) Seasons of survival: reflections of a physician with cancer. N. Engl. J. Med. 313:270-273.
14. Loescher, L. J., Welch-McCaffrey, D. & Leigh, S. A. (1989) Surviving adult cancers. Part 1: Physiologic effects. Ann. Intern. Med. 111:411-432.
15. Welch-McCaffrey, D., Hoffman, B. & Leigh, S.A. (1989) Surviving adult cancers. Part 2: Psychosocial implications. Ann. Intern. Med. 111:517-524.
16. Herold, A. H. & Roetzheim, R. G. (1992) Cancer survivors. Primary Care 19:779-791.
17. Marina, N. (1997) Long-term survivors of childhood cancer. The medical consequences of cure. Pediatr. Clin. N. Am. 44:1021-1041.
18. Blatt, J, Copeland, D. R. & Bleyer, W. A. (1997) Late effects of childhood cancer and its treatment. Pizzo, P.A. Poplack, D.G. eds. Principles and Practice of Pediatric Oncology 1997:1091-1114 J.B. Lippincott Philadelphia, PA.
19. Meadows AT, Krejmas NL, Belasco JB. The medical cost of cure: sequelae in survivors of childhood cancer. In: Van Eys J, Sullivan MP, (eds). Status of the curability of childhood cancers. New York: Raven Press, 1980;263-276.
20. Lipshultz SE, Colan SD, Gelber RD et al. Late cardiac effects of doxorubicin therapy for acute lymphoblastic leukemia in childhood. N Engl J Med, 1991;324:808-814.
21. Steinherz LJ, Steinherz PG. Cardiac failure and dysrhythmias 6-19 years after anthracycline therapy: a series of 15 patients. Med Pediatr Oncol, 1995;24:352-361.

22. van Dam FS, Schagen SB, Muller MJ. Impairment of cognitive function in women receiving adjuvant treatment for high-risk breast cancer: high-dose versus standard-dose chemotherapy. JNCI,1998;90:210-8.
23. Brezden CB, Phillips KA, Abdolell M. Cognitive function in breast cancer patients receiving adjuvant chemotherapy. J Clin Oncol, 2000;l8:2695-701.
24. Ochs J, Mulhern RK, Faircough D. Comparison of neuropsychologic function and clinical indicators of neurotoxicity in long-term survivors of childhood leukemia given cranial irradiation or parenteral methotrexate: a prospective study. J Clin Oncol, 1991;9:145 -151.
25. Meyers CA, Weitzner MA: Neurobehavioral functioning and quality of life in patients treated for cancer of the central nervous system. Current Opinion in Oncology, 1995;7:197-200.
26. Ganz PA, Greendale GA, Petersen L, Zibecchi L, Kahn B, Belin TR. Managing menopausal symptoms in breast cancer survivors: results of a randomized controlled trial. J Natl Cancer Inst, 2000;5:1054-64.
27. Greendale GA, Petersen L, Zibecchi L, Ganz PA. Factors related to sexual function in postmenopausal women with a history of breast cancer. Menopause, 2001;8:111-9.
28. Lamb MA. Effects of Cancer on the Sexuality and Fertility of Women. Seminars in Oncology Nursing, 1995;11:120-127.
29. Goodwin PJ, Ennis M, Pritchard KI et al. Risk of menopause during the first year after breast cancer diagnosis. J Clin Oncol, 1999;17:2365-2370.
30. Constine LS, Rubin P, Woolf PD et al. Hyperprolactinemia and hypothyroidism following cytotoxic therapy for central nervous system malignancies. J Clin Oncol, 1987;5:1841-1851.
31. Andrykowski MA, Curran SL, Lightner R. Off-treatment fatigue in breast cancer survivors: a controlled comparison. J of Behav Med, 1998;21:1-18.
32. Loge JH, Abrahamsen AF, Ekeberg O, Kaasa S. Hodgkin's disease survivors more fatigued than the general population. J Clin Oncol, 1999;17:253-261.
33. Bhatia S, Robison LL, Oberlin O. Breast cancer and other second neoplasms after childhood Hodgkin's disease. N Engl J Med, 1996;334:745-751.
34. Meyer TA and Mark MM. Effects of psychosocial interventions with adult cancer patients: A meta-analysis of randomized experiments. Health Psychology, 14:101-108.
35. Devine EC and Westlake SK. The effects of psychoeducational care provided to adults with cancer: meta-analysis of 116 studies. Oncol Nurs Forum,1995;22:1369-1381.
36. Ganz PA, Desmond KA, Leedham B, Rowland JH, Meyerowitz BE, Belin TR. Quality of Life in Long-term, disease-free survivors of breast cancer: a follow-up study. J Natl Cancer Inst, 2002; 94:39-49.
37. Gotay CC, Muraoka MY. Quality of life in ling-term survivors of adult-onset cancers. J Natl Cancer Inst, 1998; 90:656-67.
38. Andersen BL. Surviving Cancer. Cancer, 1994;74:1484-95.
39. Kornblith AB. Psychosocial adaptation of cancer survivors. In: Holland JC et al (eds). Psycho-Oncology. New York, Oxford University Press, 1998.
40. Schnoll RA, Malstrom M, James C, Rothman RL, Miller SM, Ridge JA, et al. Correlates of Tobacco use among smokers and recent quitters diagnosed with cancer. Patient Education Counseling, 2001;1517:1-12.
41. Stuber ML, Christakis DM, Houskamp B, Kazak AE. Post trauma symptoms in childhood leukemia survivors and their parents. Psychosomatics, 1996;37:254-261.
42. Raveis VH, Karus D, Pretter S. Correlates of anxiety among adult daughter caregivers to a parent with cancer. J Psychosoc Oncol, 1999;17:1-26.
43. Yancik R, Ganz PA, Varricchio CG, Conley B. Perspectives on comorbidity and cancer in older patients: approaches to expand the knowledge base. J Clin Oncol, 2001;19:1147-51.
44. Aziz N. Late Effects of Cancer Treatment and Follow-Up Care Needs Among Cancer Survivors. Invited Commentary and Foreword. AJN; 2006; 106 Suppl 3:3.
45. Day RW: Future need for more cancer research. J Am Diet Assoc 98: 523, 1998.
46. Brown BW, Brauner C, Minnotte MC: Noncancer deaths in white adult cancer patients. JNCI 85: 979-997, 1993.
47. Travis LB: Therapy-associated solid tumors. Acta Oncol 41:323-333, 2002.
48. Bergstrom A, Pisani P, Tenet V. Overweight as an avoidable cause of cancer in Europe. Intern J Cancer 91:421-430, 2001.
49. World Health Organization: IARC Handbook of Cancer Prevention (ISSN 1027-5622) Vol 6, 2002.
50. Chlebowski RT, Aiello E, McTiernan A. Weight loss in breast cancer patient management. J Clin Oncol 20,1128-1143, 2002.
51. Nuver J, Smit AJ, Postma A: The metabolic syndrome in long-term cancer survivors, an important target for secondary measures. Cancer Treat Rev 28:195–214, 2002.
52. Freedland SJ, Aronson WJ, Kane CJ. Impact of obesity on biochemical control after radical prostatectomy for clinically localized prostate cancer: a report by the Shared Equal Access Regional Cancer Hospital database study group. J Clin Oncol 22:446-453, 2004.
53. Argiles JM Lopez-Soriano FJ. Insulin and cancer. Intern J Oncol 18: 683-687, 2001.
54. Bines J, Gradishar WJ. Primary care issues for the breast cancer survivor. Compr Ther 23: 605-611,1997.
55. Yoshikawa T, Noguchi Y, Doi C. Insulin resistance in patients with cancer: relationships with tumor site, tumor stage, body-weight loss, acute-phase response, and energy expenditure. Nutr 17: 590-593, 2001.
56. Balkau B, Kahn HS, Courbon D. Paris Prospective Study. Hyperinsulinemia predicts fatal liver cancer but is inversely associated with fatal cancer at some other sites: the Paris Prospective Study. Diabetes Care 24:843-849, 2001.
57. Lamont EB, Christakis NA, Lauderdale DS. Favorable cardiac risk among elderly breast carcinoma survivors. Cancer 98: 2-10, 2003.
58. Hull MC, Morris CG, Pepine CJ. Valvular dysfunction and carotid, subclavian, and coronary artery disease in survivors of Hodgkin lymphoma treated with radiation therapy. JAMA 290:2831-2837, 2003.
59. Lamont EB, Lauderdale DS. Low risk of hip fracture among elderly breast cancer survivors. Ann Epidemiol 13:698-703, 2003.
60. Newcomb PA, Trentham-Dietz A, Egan KM. Fracture history and risk of breast and endometrial cancer. Am J Epidemiol.153:1071-1078, 2001.

61 van der Klift M, de Laet CE, Coebergh JW. Bone mineral density and the risk of breast cancer: the Rotterdam Study. Bone 32:211-216, 2003.

62 Zmuda JM, Cauley JA, Ljung BM. Study of Osteoporotic Fractures Research Group. Bone mass and breast cancer risk in older women: differences by stage at diagnosis. JNCI 93:930-936, 2001.

63 Schultz PN, Beck ML, Stava C. Health profiles in 5836 long-term cancer survivors. Intern J Cancer 104: 488-495, 2003.

64 Diamond TH, Higano CS, Smith MR. Osteoporosis in men with prostate carcinoma receiving androgen-deprivation therapy: recommendations for diagnosis and therapies. Cancer 100:892-899, 2004.

65 Ko CY, Maggard M, Livingston EH. Evaluating health utility in patients with melanoma, breast cancer, colon cancer, and lung cancer: a nationwide, population-based assessment. J Surg Res 114:1-5, 2003.

66 Garman KS, Pieper CF, Seo P. Function in elderly cancer survivors depends on comorbidities. J Gerontol A Biol Sci Med Sci 58: M1119-M1124, 2003.

67 Hewitt M, Rowland JH, Yancik R: Cancer survivors in the U.S.: age, health and disability. J Gerontol Biol Sci Med Sci 58:82-91, 2003.

68 Ashing-Giwa K, Ganz PA, Petersen L: Quality of life of African-American and white long term breast carcinoma survivors. Cancer 85:418-426, 1999.

69 Baker F, Haffer S, Denniston M: Health-related quality of life of cancer and noncancer patients in Medicare managed care. Cancer 97:674-681, 2003.

70 Chirikos TN, Russell-Jacobs A, Jacobsen PB: Functional impairment and the economic consequences of female breast cancer. Womens Health 36:1-20, 2002.

71 Ness KK, Mertens AC, Hudson MM, Wall MM, Leisenring WM, Oeffinger KC, Sklar CA, Robison LL, Gurney JG. Limitations on physical performance and daily activities among long-term survivors of childhood cancer. Ann Intern Med. 2005 Nov 1;143(9):639-47

72 Oeffinger KC, Mertens AC, Sklar CA, Kawashima T, Hudson MM, Meadows AT, et al. Childhood Cancer Survivor Study. Chronic health conditions in adult survivors of childhood cancer. N Engl J Med. 2006 Oct 12;355(15):1572-82.

73 Michael YL, Kawachi I, Berkman LF, Holmes MD, Colditz GA. The persistent impact of breast carcinoma on functional health status: prospective evidence from the Nurses' Health Study. Cancer. 2000 Dec 1;89(11):2176-86.

74 Kroenke CH, Rosner B, Chen WY, Kawachi I, Colditz GA, Holmes MD. Functional impact of breast cancer by age at diagnosis. J Clin Oncol. 2004 May 15;22(10):1849-56.

75 Michael YL, Berkman LF, Colditz GA, Holmes MD, Kawachi I. Social networks and health-related quality of life in breast cancer survivors: a prospective study. J Psychosom Res. 2002 May;52(5):285-93.

76 Ahles TA, Saykin AJ, Noll WW, Furstenberg CT, Guerin S, Cole B, Mott LA. The relationship of APOE genotype to neuropsychological performance in long-term cancer survivors treated with standard dose chemotherapy. Psychooncology. 2003 Sep;12(6):612-9.

77 Lipshultz SE. Exposure to anthracyclines during childhood causes cardiac injury. Semin Oncol. 2006 Jun;33(3 Suppl 8):S8-14.

78 Lipshultz SE, Vlach SA, Lipsitz SR, Sallan SE, Schwartz ML, Colan SD. Cardiac changes associated with growth hormone therapy among children treated with anthracyclines. Pediatrics. 2005 Jun;115(6):1613-22.

79 Lipshultz SE, Rifai N, Dalton VM, Levy DE, Silverman LB, Lipsitz SR, et al. The effect of dexrazoxane on myocardial injury in doxorubicin-treated children with acute lymphoblastic leukemia. N Engl J Med. 2004 Jul 8;351(2):145-53.

80 Adams MJ, Lipsitz SR, Colan SD, Tarbell NJ, Treves ST, Diller L, et al. Cardiovascular status in long-term survivors of Hodgkin's disease treated with chest radiotherapy. J Clin Oncol. 2004 Aug 1;22(15):3139-48.

81 Ahles TA, Saykin AJ, Furstenberg CT, Cole B, Mott LA, Titus-Ernstoff L, et al. Quality of life of long-term survivors of breast cancer and lymphoma treated with standard-dose chemotherapy or local therapy. J Clin Oncol. 2005 Jul 1;23(19):4399-405.

82 Blatt, J., Bercu, B. B. & Gillin, J. C. (1984) Reduced pulsatile growth hormone secretion in children after therapy for acute lymphoblastic leukemia. J. Pediatr. 104:182-186.

83 Ogilvy-Stuart, A. L., Clayton, P. E. & Shalet, S. M. (1994) Cranial irradiation and early puberty. J. Clin. Endocrinol Metab. 78:1282-1286.

84 Didi, M., Didcock, E. & Davies, H. A. (1995) High incidence of obesity in young adults after treatment of acute lymphoblastic leukemia in childhood. J. Pediatr. 127:63-67.

85 Sklar, C, Mertens, A. & Walter, A. (1993) Final height after treatment for childhood acute lymphoblastic leukemia: comparison of no cranial irradiation with 1,800 and 2,400 centigrays of cranial irradiation. J. Pediatr. 123:59-64.

86 Furst, C. J., Lundell, M. & Ahlback, S. O. (1989) Breast hypoplasia following irradiation of the female breast in infancy and early childhood. Acta Oncol. 28:519-523.

87 Haupt, R., Fears, T. R. & Robeson, L. L. (1994) Educational attainment in long-term survivors of childhood acute lymphoblastic leukemia. J. Am. Med. Assoc. 272:1427-1432.

88 Ochs, J., Mulhern, R. K. & Faircough, D. (1991) Comparison of neuropsychologic function and clinical indicators of neurotoxicity in long-term survivors of childhood leukemia given cranial irradiation or parenteral methotrexate: a prospective study. J. Clin. Oncol. 9:145-151.

89 Kreuser, E. D., Hetzel, W. D. & Heit, W. (1988) Reproductive and endocrine gonadal functions in adults following multidrug chemotherapy for acute lymphoblastic or undifferentiated leukemia. J. Clin. Oncol. 6:588-595.

90 Sklar CA, Mertens AC, Mitby P, Whitton J, Stovall M, Kasper C, et al. Premature menopause in survivors of childhood cancer: a report from the childhood cancer survivor study. J Natl Cancer Inst. 2006 Jul 5;98(13):890-6.

91 Chemaitilly W, Mertens AC, Mitby P, Whitton J, Stovall M, Yasui Y, et al. Acute ovarian failure in the childhood cancer survivor study. J Clin Endocrinol Metab. 2006 May;91(5):1723-8. Epub 2006 Feb 21.

92 Shahin, M. S. & Puscheck, E. (1998) Reproductive sequelae of cancer treatment. Obstet. Gynecol. Clin. N. Am. 25:423-433.

93 Greendale, G. A., Petersen, L., Zibecchi, L. & Ganz, P. A. (2001) Factors related to sexual function in postmeno-

pausal women with a history of breast cancer. Menopause 8:111-119.
94. Deimling GT, Sterns S, Bowman KF, Kahana B. The health of older-adult, long-term cancer survivors. Cancer Nurs. 2005 Nov-Dec;28(6):415-24.
95. Aziz N. Follow-up Care for Cancer Survivors: Developing the Evidence Base. Invited Commentary. Annals of Family Medicine; July 2004.
96. Kattlove H, Winn RJ: Ongoing Care of Patients After Primary Treatment for Their Cancer. CA Cancer J Clin 2003 53:172-196, 2003.
97. Robison LL: Cancer survivorship: Unique opportunities for research. Cancer Epidemiol Biomarkers Prev 13:1093, 2004.
98. Eshelman D, Landier W, Sweeney T, Hester AL, Forte K, Darling J, et al. Facilitating care for childhood cancer survivors: integrating children's oncology group long-term follow-up guidelines and health links in clinical practice. J Pediatr Oncol Nurs, 2004; 21:271-80.
99. Eshelman D, Landier W, Sweeney T, Hester AL, Forte K, Darling J, et al. Facilitating care for childhood cancer survivors: integrating children's oncology group long-term follow-up guidelines and health links in clinical practice. J Pediatr Oncol Nurs. 2004 Sep-Oct;21(5):271-80.
100. Yabroff KR. Burden of illness in cancer survivors: findings from a population-based national sample. J Natl Cancer Inst 2004;96(17):1322-30.
101. Earle CC, Neville BA. Under use of necessary care among cancer survivors. Cancer 2004;101(8):1712-9.
102. Deimling GT. Cancer survivorship and psychological distress in later life. Psychooncology 2002;11(6):479-94.
103. Ferrell BR, Hassey Dow K. Quality of life among long-term cancer survivors. Oncology (Williston Park) 1997;11(4):565-8, 71; discussion 72, 75-6.
104. From Cancer Patient to Cancer Survivor: Lost in Transition. Hewitt M, Greenfield S, and Stovall E, eds. National Academies Press, Washington D.C., 2005.
105. Childhood Cancer Survivorship: Improving Care and Quality of Life. Hewitt M, Weiner S, and Simone J, eds. National Academies Press Washington D.C. 2003
106. Taylor A, Blacklay A, Davies H, Douglas C, Jenney M, Wallace H, Levitt G Long-term follow-up of survivors of childhood cancer in the UK. Pediatr Blood Cancer. 2004;42(2):161-8.
107. Wallace WH, Blacklay A, Eiser C, Davies H, Hawkins M, Levitt G, Jenney M (2001) Developing strategies for long-term follow-up of survivors of childhood cancer BMJ 323: 271-274.
108. Birgisson H, Pahlman L, Gunnarson U, Glimelius B, The Swedish Rectal Cancer Trial Group. Adverse effects of preoperative radiation therapy for rectal cancer: Long-term follow-up of the Swedish Rectal Cancer Trial. J Clin Oncol 2005;23:8697_705.
109. Travis LB, Rabkin CS, Brown LM, Allan JM, Blanche PA, Ambrosone CB, et al. Cancer survivorship-Genetic susceptibility and second primary cancers: Research strategies and recommendations. J Natl Cancer Inst 2006; 98:15_25.
110. Oldenburg J, Kraggerud SM, Cvancarova M, Lothe RA, Fossa SD. Cisplatin-induced long-term hearing impairment is associated with specific glutathione-s-transferase genotypes in testicular cancer survivors. In. 2006.
111. Andreassen CN. Can risk of radiotherapy-induced normal tissue complications be predicted from genetic profiles? Acta Oncol 2005; 44:801_5.
112. Nord C, Ganz PA, Aziz NM, Fossa SD. Long term follow up of cancer survivors in the Nordic Countries. Acta Oncologica, In Press, 2007.
113. Hudson MM. A model for care across the cancer continuum. Supplement to Cancer 2005; 104:2638_42.
114. Travis LB. Therapy-associated solid tumors. Acta Oncol 2002; 41:323_33.
115. Pakilit AT, Kahn BA, Petersen L, Abraham LS, Greendale GA, Ganz PA. Making effective use of tumour registries for cancer survivorship research. Cancer 2001; 92:1305_14.
116. Skinner R WWLG, UK Children's Cancer Study Group Late Effects Group. Long-term follow-up of people who have survived cancer during childhood. Lancet Oncol 2006;7:489_98.
117. Nord C, Mykletun A, Fossa SD. Cancer patients' awareness about their diagnosis: A population-based study. J Publ Health Med 2003; 25:313_7
118. Nord C, Mykletun A, Thorsen L, Bjøro T, Fossa SD. Selfreported health and use of health care services in long-term cancer survivors. Int J Cancer 2005; 114:307_16
119. Natsch S, van der Meer JWM. The role of clinical guidelines, policies and stewardship. J Hospital Infect 2003; 53:172_6.
120. Landier W, Bhatia S, Eshelman DA, Forte KJ, Sweeney T, Hester AL, et al. Development of risk-based guidelines for pediatric cancer survivors: The Children's Oncology Group Long-Term Follow-Up Guidelines from the Children's Oncology Group Late Effects Committee and Nursing Discipline. J Clin Oncol 2004; 22:4979_90.
121. Hudson MM. A model for care across the cancer continuum. Supplement to Cancer 2005; 104:2638_42.
122. Friedman DL, Freyer DR, Levitt GA. Models of care for survivors of childhood cancer. Pediatr Blood Cancer 2006; 46:159_68.
123. Oeffinger KC, McCabe MS. Models for delivering survivorship care. J Clin Oncol 2006; 24:5117_24.

Subject Index

A

adhesion molecule 21
adriamycin 104, 115
adverse late effect 99, 101
Akt pathway 26
amifostine 13, 64
ANCOVA 93
angiogenesis 20
angiotensin 70, 73
– II 15
– converting enzyme (ACE) 15, 20, 69
– blocker 74
– inhibitors 72
angiotensinogen 69
ANOVA 91, 96
anthracycline 50, 52, 53, 115
aortic stenosis 52
APOE 115
apoptosis 15
arrhythmia 49, 53, 55
ASCO 118
atrioventricular nodal bradycardia 52
autonomic dysfunction 49
axillary node metastases 50
azotemia 71

B

basic fibroblast growth factor (bFGF) 25, 26, 64
bFGF, see basic fibroblast growth factor
biodosimetry 14
biologic continuum 101
blood vessel 19
BMT, see bone marrow transplantation
bone marrow transplantation (BMT) 71
– nephropathy syndrome 74
– TBI-based 74
bradykinin pathway 71
brain
– atrophy 42
– injury 42
– – radiation-induced 42
breast cancer 39, 41, 48, 49, 52, 92, 93, 114, 115

C

C. elegans 14
cancer
– comorbidity 117
– early detection 110
– long-term toxicity 122
– second cancer 117
– survivorship
– – care plan 123
– – community care 124
– – comorbidity 113
– – domains 125
– – follow-up 117
– – IOM report 118
– – late effects 111
– – long-term 110, 112
– – paradigm 111
– – phases 110
– – research 109
– treatment 112
– – guidelines for follow-up care 119
cancer-related fatigue (CRF) 91, 97
captopril 70–72
carcinogen 77
carcinogenesis 13
carcinoma
– of the cervix 78
– of the prostate 78
cardiac disease, radiation-induced 41
cardiomyopathy 50, 55, 56, 116
– different types 51
cardiovascular disease (CVD) 48, 114
– radiation-induced 49
– screening 48
Centers for Medical Countermeasures against Radiation (CMCR) 15
chemotherapy 115
– fatigue 92
– late effects 120
childhood cancer 1
chylothorax 54
cisplatinum 104
coagulation 20
collagen
– release 28
– type III 26, 27
Common Toxicity Criteria (CTC) V3.0 100

Community Clinical Oncology Program (CCOP) 92
competing
– plan 85
– treatment 83
coronary
– artery disease 49, 116
– heart disease 55
CRF, see cancer-related fatigue
CTC, see Common Toxicity Criteria
CVD, see cardiovascular disease
cytokine 15, 21, 24, 35
– cascade 101
– pathway 64
cytosine arabinoside 115
cytoskeleton (F-actin filaments) 21

D

decision analysis 83
decreased functional status 114
depression 95, 97
dexrazoxane 116
diabetes 114
diabetic nephropathy 71
diastolic dysfunction 50
dobutamine 56
Doppler echocardiography 56
dose-volume constraints 85
duration factor 85

E

echocardiography 56
effect time course 99
electron spin resonance (ESR) 63
enalapril 72
endocarditis 52
endothelial cell (EC) 19
endothelium 19
EORTC, see European Organisation for Research on Treatment of Cancer
epithelial growth factor 15
E-selectin 25, 26
ESR, see electron spin resonance
European Organisation for Research on Treatment of Cancer (EORTC)
– RTOG/EORTC scales 99, 100
excess relative risk 80

F

F-actin filaments 21
Fajardo, Luis 12
fatigue 95
– based on age 95
– based on gender 96
– cancer-related 91

– severity of symptoms 94, 95, 97
– subset analyses 96
fibrinolysis 21
fibrosis 23, 24, 27, 28
– of the conduction pathways 52
– of the myocardium 50
– pulmonary 25
fluorodeoxyglucose (FDG) uptake 42
follow-up care 118
– research 122
Framingham Heart Study 52

G

gene induction 13
genetic disorder 77
glioma 42
global toxicity grade 106
guidelines 3
– development 123
– dissemination 9
– interactive 6
– patient-specific tools 7
– revisions 5
– updates 5
– web-based 6
health care utilization 113
health-related quality of life 113
heart
– block 52
– disease, radiation-induced
– – risk factors 54
– injury 41
– transplantation 56
hematopoietic cytokine 15
herceptin 116
Hodgkin's disease/lymphoma 41, 43, 48, 115, 116
hydrogen peroxide 62, 63
hydroxyl radical 62
hyperinsulinemia 114
hypertension 71
hypothyroidism 54
hypoxia 61, 62

I

ICAM-1, see intracellular adhesion molecule-1
improved nuclear device (IND) 11
IMRT, see intensity-modulated radiation therapy
IND, see improved nuclear device
inflammatory response 35, 62
intensity-modulated radiation therapy (IMRT) 79
– dynamic 80
– step and shoot method 80
intracellular adhesion molecule-1 (ICAM-1) 25–29
ischemia 52

J

Japanese A-bomb survivor 78

K

Kallman, Robert
Kaplan, Henry S. 12
Karnofsky performance index 93
kidney 69
– microsomes 73

L

late effect 1, 2
– follow-up care 120
– normal tissue (LENT) 99, 100, 103
– physiologic 115
LDL cholesterol 55
LENT, see late effects normal tissue
linear accelerator 12
local tumor control 86
losartan 70
lumpectomy 50
lung
– cancer
– – dose-effect relation 40
– – patients 83
– – SPECT perfusion images 40
– fibrosis 38
– injury, radiation-induced 38
– malignant lymphoma 39
lymphocyte 65

M

macrophage 62, 65
– NADPH oxidase 61
magnetic resonance imaging (MRI) 40
malignant neoplasm 115
mastectomy 48, 49
maximal oxygen consumption 56
mediastinal
– fibrosis 56
– radiation 48
medical countermeasures 11
metabolic syndrome-associated disease 113
methotrexate 115
micronucleus 32
mitigator 14
monocyte 62
MRI, see magnetic resonance imaging
mucoepidermoid carcinoma 43
multi-disciplinary task forces 4
myocardial
– disease 55
– fibrosis 49, 52

N

National Institute for Allergy and Infectious Diseases (NIAID) 14
neck cancer 92
nephropathy 71
NF-κB 24, 26
non-renal tissue 73
non-severe grade 86
non-small-cell lung cancer (NSCLC)
normal tissue 11
– complication probability (NTCP) 84
– – QALY 84
– hypoxia-mediated chronic injury 61
– radiation-induced injury 37, 43
– risks 88
– TNM toxicity taxonomy 99
NSCLC, see non-small-cell lung cancer
NTCP, see normal tissue complication probability
nuclear warface 12
numerical taxonomy 101, 102

O

obesity 113
operational taxonomic unit (OTU) 102, 104
osteoporosis 114, 116
out-of-field
– damage 34
– effect 33
oxidative stress 63

P

paired t-test 95
passport for care 6, 9
patient education 4
patient-rated quality 87
PDGF, see platelet-derived growth factor
PDSA (plan-do-study-act) cycle 123
pentoxyfylline 15
pericarditis 49, 53, 55
phosphatidylinositol-3 kinase (PI3K) 26, 27
– PI3K/Akt inhibition 28
PI3K, see phosphatidylinositol-3 kinase
plan scoring 87
plasminogen activator 20
platelet adhesion 20
platelet-derived growth factor (PDGF) 25, 26
pleomorphic adenoma 43
pneumocytes type II 24, 28
pneumonitis 23–28, 86
post-mastectomy radiation therapy (PMRT) 50
premature menopause 116
proliferating cell nuclear antigen (PCNA) 72
prostate cancer 92, 93
proteinuria 71, 72
proton 81

pulmonary
- fibrosis 25
- function test 56

Q

QALY, *see* quality-adjusted life years
quality of life 113, 118
quality-adjusted life years (QALY) 83

R

RABRAT 14
radiation 19
- lung injury 38
- nephropathy 71, 72
- pneumopathy 73
- protection 13
- therapy
- - cardiotoxicity 49
- - fatigue 92
Radiation Therapy Oncology Group (RTOG) 74
- RTOG/EORTC scales 99, 100
radiation-induced
- brain injury 42
- cardiac disease 41
- cardiovascular disease (CVD) 48, 114
- heart disease 54
- lung injury 38
- normal tissue injury 37, 43
- sarcoma 79
- second cancer/carcinoma 79
radiological dispersion device (RDD) 11
Radiological Events Medical Management (REMM) 16
radionuclide
- myocardial perfusion 56
- ventriculography 50, 56
radiotherapy
- combination with chemotherapy 89
- late effects 120
ramipril 70, 70
RAS, *see* renin-angiotensin system
RDD, *see* radiological dispersion device
reactive
- nitroxyl species (RNS) 35
- oyxgen species (ROS) 35, 62
recombinant human keratinocyte growth factor (rhuKGF) 65
relative risk categories 88
renin-angiotensin system (RAS) 69
rhuKGF, *see* recombinant human keratinocyte growth factor
RNS, *see* reactive nitroxyl species
ROS, *see* reactive oxygen species
RTOG, *see* Radiation Therapy Oncology Group

S

salivary glands 42
- radiation injury 42

sarcoma, radiation-induced 79
scanning beam 81
scintigraphy 41, 43
scoliosis 53
screening 1
- recommendations 2, 3
second
- cancer/carcinoma 81
- malignancy 77, 81
SEER program 78
selectin 28
serum
- creatinine 74
- renin 72
shortness of breath 95, 97
sialadenitis 42
sick sinus syndrome 52
single photon emission computed tomography (SPECT) 39, 50
- perfusion images
- - heart injury 41
- - lung cancer 40
SOD, *see* superoxide dismutase
SOMA, *see* subjective objective management analytic
SOMA/LENT system 43
SPECT, *see* single photon emission computed tomography
state of health 84
statin 64, 65
step and shoot method 80
subjective objective management analytic (SOMA) 99
summary toxicity grade 105
superoxide 62
- dismutase (SOD) 63, 64
symptom
- inventory (SI) 92
- severity data 94

T

tachycardia 53
taxonomy 101
TBI, *see* total-body irradiation
Tc-99m sestamibi scintigraphy 41
TCP, *see* tumor control probability
teprotide 70
TGF, *see* transforming growth factor
thalidomide 64
therapeutic exposure 3
thoracic
- duct fibrosis 53
- radiation 38, 47, 48
tissue hypoxia 61
TNM
- language 103
- taxonomy 99
- toxicity 99
total-body irradiation (TBI) 71, 73
transforming growth factor (TGF) 24
- TGF-α 26
- TGF-β 15, 28, 62, 64

treatment
- late complications 2
- plan 83
troponin 116
tumor
- control probability (TCP) 84
- necrosis factor alpha (TNF-α) 24–26, 64

U

uncomplicated tumor control probability (UTCP) 84
- classic formula 86
- QALY-weighted 83, 85
University of Rochester Cancer Center (URCC) 92
- symptom inventory 92
UTCP, see uncomplicated tumor control probability
uterine cancer 97
utility factor 85

V

valvular disease 49, 52, 55

vascular
- endothelial growth factor (VEGF) 62, 64
- permeability 21
VEGF, see vascular endothelial growth factor
vinca alkaloid 115
volume
- effect 35
- - apex 33
- - base 33
- - irradiating different volumes 32, 33
- - lung region 33
- - out-of-field effect 33
- - regional effects 32
- irradiation 33

Y

yeast 14

Z

Zebrafish 14

List of Contributors

M. JACOB ADAMS, MD, MPH
Department of Community and Preventive Medicine
Division of Epidemiology
University of Rochester School of Medicine and Dentistry
601 Elmwood Avenue, Box 644
Rochester, NY 14642
USA

MITCHELL STEVEN ANSCHER, MD
Department of Radiation Oncology
Virginia Commonwealth University Medical Center
Box 980058
401 College St.
Richmond, VA 23298-0058
USA

NOREEN M. AZIZ, MD, PhD, MPH
Senior Program Director
Office of Cancer Survivorship
Division of Cancer Control & Population Sciences
National Cancer Institute, Bethesda, MD
6116 Executive Boulevard
Bethesda, MD 20892
USA

SMITA BHATIA, MD
City of Hope National Medical Center
Division of Pediatrics
Chair, Division of Cancer Prevention & Control
1500 East Duarte Road, MO8B4
Duarte, CA 91010
USA

CHRISTOPHER BOLE, MA
Department of Radiation Oncology
James P. Wilmot Cancer Center
University of Rochester School of Medicine and Dentistry
Behavioral Medicine Unit
Box 704, 601 Elmwood Ave.
Rochester, NY 14642
USA

DAVID J. BRENNER, Dphil, DSc
Center for Radiological Research
Columbia University Medical Center
College of Physicians & Surgeons
630 W. 168th St., P&S 11-230
New York, NY 10032
USA

J. MARTIN BROWN, PhD
Professor of Radiation Oncology – Radiation Biology
Department of Radiation Oncology
Stanford University School of Medicine
269 Campus Drive West
CCSR South, Room 1255
Stanford, CA 94305
USA

ERIC P. COHEN, MD
Department of Medicine
Nephrology Division
Medical College of Wisconsin
9200 W. Wisconsin Ave.
Milwaukee, WI 53226
USA

C. NORMAN COLEMAN, MD
Associate Director, Radiation Research Program
EPN/Room 6014
6130 Executive Blvd.
Bethesda, MD 20892
USA

LOUIS S. CONSTINE, MD
Professor of Radiation Oncology and Pediatrics
Vice Chair, Department of Radiation Oncology
Departments of Radiation Oncology and Pediatrics
University of Rochester
School of Medicine and Dentistry
601 Elmwood Avenue, Box 647
Rochester, NY 14642
USA

LUIS FELIPE FAJARDO L-G, MD
Professor, Department of Pathology
Stanford University School of Medicine
and Veterans Affairs Medical Center
3801 Miranda Ave.
Palo Alto, CA 94304
USA

COLMAR FIGUEROA-MOSELEY, PhD
Department of Radiation Oncology
James P. Wilmot Cancer Center
University of Rochester School of Medicine and Dentistry
Behavioral Medicine Unit
Box 704, 601 Elmwood Ave.
Rochester, NY 14642
USA

MICHAEL FORDIS, MD
Director, Center for Collaborative and
Interactive Technologies
Senior Associate Dean and Director
Office of Continuing Medical Education
Baylor College of Medicine
Mailing Address:
One Baylor Plaza, MS155
Houston, TX 77030
USA

OLIVIER GAYOU, PhD
Department of Radiation Oncology
Allegheny General Hospital
320 East North Avenue
Pittsburgh, Pennsylvania 15212
USA

ERIC J. HALL, Dphil, DSc, FACR, FRCR
Center for Radiological Research
Columbia University Medical Center
College of Physicians & Surgeons
630 W. 168th St., P&S 11-230
New York, NY 10032
USA

DENNIS E. HALLAHAN, MD
Department of Radiation Oncology
Vanderbilt University Medical Center
1301 22nd Ave South
B-902 The Vanderbilt Clinic
Nashville, TN 37232
USA

RICHARD P. HILL, PhD
Research Division, Ontario Cancer Institute
Princess Margaret Hospital
University Health Network
Departments of Medical Biophysics and
Radiation Oncology
University of Toronto
610 University Ave.
Toronto, Ontario M5G 2M9
Canada

MAARTEN HOFMAN, MS
Department of Radiation Oncology
James P. Wilmot Cancer Center
University of Rochester School of Medicine and Dentistry
Behavioral Medicine Unit
Box 704, 601 Elmwood Ave.
Rochester, NY 14642
USA

MARC HOROWITZ, MD
Professor of Pediatrics
Texas Children's Cancer Center
Baylor College of Medicine
6621 Fannin Street, CC 1410.00
Houston, TX 77030
USA

MELISSA M. HUDSON, MD
Member, Department of Oncology
Director, Cancer Survivorship Division Medicine
St. Jude Children's Research Hospital
332 North Lauderdale; Mailstop 735
Memphis, TN 38105-2794
USA

MELISSA M. JOINES, MD
Department of Medicine and Radiation Oncology
Medical College of Wisconsin
9200 W. Wisconsin Ave.
Milwaukee, WI 53226
USA

MARALYN E. KAUFMAN, PhD
Department of Radiation Oncology
James P. Wilmot Cancer Center
University of Rochester School of Medicine
and Dentistry
Behavioral Medicine Unit
Box 704, 601 Elmwood Ave.
Rochester, NY 14642
USA

MOHAMMED A. KHAN, MD
Research Division, Ontario Cancer Institute
Princess Margaret Hospital
University Health Network
610 University Ave.
Toronto, Ontario M5G 2M9
Canada

ZAFER KOCAK, MD
Department of Radiation Oncology
Duke University Medical Center
Box 3085
Durham, NC 27710
and
Department of Radiation Oncology
Trakya University Hospital
22030 Edirnne
Turkey

WENDY LANDIER, RN, MSN, CPNP, CPON
City of Hope National Medical Center
1500 E. Duarte Rd., MOB-4
Duarte, CA 91010-3000
USA

AIMEE R. LANGAN, MD
Research Division, Ontario Cancer Institute
Princess Margaret Hospital
University Health Network
Departments of Medical Biophysics and
Radiation Oncology
University of Toronto
610 University Ave.
Toronto, Ontario M5G 2M9
Canada

STEVEN E. LIPSHULTZ, MD
Professor, Department of Pediatrics
University of Miami School of Medicine
P.O. Box 016820
Miami, FL 33101
USA

LAWRENCE B. MARKS, MD
Professor, Department of Radiation Oncology
Duke University Medical Center
P.O. Box 3085
Durham, NC 27710
USA

ANNA T. MEADOWS, MD
Professor of Pediatrics
University of Pennsylvania
Children's Hospital of Philadelphia
Division of Oncology
34th Street & Civic Center Blvd.
Philadelphia, PA 19104
USA

MOYED MIFTEN, PhD
Department of Radiation Oncology
Allegheny General Hospital
Associate Professor, Drexel University College of Medicine
320 East North Avenue
Pittsburgh, Pennsylvania 15212
USA

GARY R. MORROW, PhD, MS
Professor of Radiation Oncology
Professor of Psychiatry
Director, URCC CCOP Research Base
Department of Radiation Oncology
James P. Wilmot Cancer Center
University of Rochester School of Medicine and Dentistry
Behavioral Medicine Unit
Box 704, 601 Elmwood Ave.
Rochester, NY 14642
USA

JOHN E. MOULDER, PhD
Professor of Radiation Oncology
Director, Center for Medical Countermeasures Against
Radialogicol Terrorisma
Medical College of Wisconsin
8701 Watertown Plank Road
Milwaukee, WI 53226
USA

KAREN M. MUSTIAN, PhD
Department of Radiation Oncology
James P. Wilmot Cancer Center
University of Rochester School of Medicine and Dentistry
Behavioral Medicine Unit
Box 704, 601 Elmwood Ave.
Rochester, NY 14642
USA

KEVIN CHARLES OEFFINGER, MD
Member, Department of Pediatrics
Memorial Sloan-Kettering Cancer Center
Department of Pediatrics
1275 York Ave
Howard #1109
New York, NY 10021
USA

PAUL OKUNIEFF, MD
Philip Rubin Professor of Radiation Oncology
Chair, Department of Radiation Oncology
University Rochester School of Medicine and Dentristry
601 Elmwood Avenue, Box 647
Rochester, NY 14642
USA

DAVID S. PARDA, MD
Department of Radiation Oncology
Allegheny General Hospital
Associate Professor, Drexel University
College of Medicine
320 East North Avenue
Pittsburgh, Pennsylvania 15212
USA

DAVID POPLACK, MD
Professor of Pediatrics
Texas Children's Cancer Center
Baylor College of Medicine
6621 Fannin Street
CC 1410.00
Houston, TX 77030
USA

ROBERT G. PROSNITZ, MD, MPH
Department of Radiation Oncology
Duke University Medical Center
P.O. Box 3085
Durham, North Carolina 27710
USA

JOSEPH A. ROSCOE, PhD
Department of Radiation Oncology
James P. Wilmot Cancer Center
University of Rochester School of
Medicine and Dentistry
Behavioral Medicine Unit
Box 704, 601 Elmwood Ave.
Rochester, NY 14642
USA

PHILIP RUBIN, MD
Professor Emeritus
Chair Emeritus
Department of Radiation Oncology
James P. Wilmot Cancer Center
University of Rochester School of Medicine and Dentistry
601 Elmwood Avenue, Box 647
Rochester, NY 14642
USA

LALITHA SHANKAR, MD, PhD
Biomedical Imaging Program
National Cancer Institute
EPN, Room 6070
6130 Executive Blvd.
Rockville, MD 20892-7412
USA

CHARLES SKLAR, MD
Member, Department of Pediatrics
Memorial Sloan Kettering Cancer Center
Department of Pediatrics
1275 York Avenue, Box 151
New York, NY 10021
USA

DANIEL C. SULLIVAN, MD, PhD
Biomedical Imaging Program
National Cancer Institute
EPN, Room 6070
6130 Executive Blvd.
Rockville, MD 20892-7412
USA

JAKE VANDYK, MD
Radiation Treatment Program
London Regional Cancer Program
London Health Sciences Centre
790, Commissioners Rd.
London, Ontario, N6A 4L6
Canada

ZELJKO VUYASKOVIC, MD, PhD
Department of Radiation Oncology
Duke University Medical Center
Box 3085 DUMC
Durham, NC 27710
USA

CHRISTOPHER D. WILLEY, MD, PhD
Department of Radiation Oncology
Vanderbilt University Medical Center
1301 22nd Ave South
B-902 The Vanderbilt Clinic
Nashville, TN 37232
USA

IVAN W.T. YEUNG, MD
Radiation Medicine Department
Princess Margaret Hospital
University Health Network
610 University Ave.
Toronto, Ontario M5G 2M9
Canada

MEDICAL RADIOLOGY Diagnostic Imaging and Radiation Oncology
Titles in the series already published

RADIATION ONCOLOGY

Lung Cancer
Edited by C.W. Scarantino

Innovations in Radiation Oncology
Edited by H. R. Withers
and L. J. Peters

**Radiation Therapy
of Head and Neck Cancer**
Edited by G. E. Laramore

**Gastrointestinal Cancer –
Radiation Therapy**
Edited by R.R. Dobelbower, Jr.

**Radiation Exposure
and Occupational Risks**
Edited by E. Scherer, C. Streffer,
and K.-R. Trott

**Radiation Therapy of Benign Diseases
A Clinical Guide**
S. E. Order and S. S. Donaldson

**Interventional Radiation
Therapy Techniques – Brachytherapy**
Edited by R. Sauer

Radiopathology of Organs and Tissues
Edited by E. Scherer, C. Streffer,
and K.-R. Trott

**Concomitant Continuous Infusion
Chemotherapy and Radiation**
Edited by M. Rotman
and C. J. Rosenthal

**Intraoperative Radiotherapy –
Clinical Experiences and Results**
Edited by F. A. Calvo, M. Santos,
and L.W. Brady

**Radiotherapy of Intraocular
and Orbital Tumors**
Edited by W. E. Alberti and
R. H. Sagerman

**Interstitial and Intracavitary
Thermoradiotherapy**
Edited by M. H. Seegenschmiedt
and R. Sauer

**Non-Disseminated Breast Cancer
Controversial Issues in Management**
Edited by G. H. Fletcher and S.H. Levitt

**Current Topics in
Clinical Radiobiology of Tumors**
Edited by H.-P. Beck-Bornholdt

**Practical Approaches to
Cancer Invasion and Metastases
A Compendium of Radiation
Oncologists' Responses to 40 Histories**
Edited by A. R. Kagan with the
Assistance of R. J. Steckel

Radiation Therapy in Pediatric Oncology
Edited by J. R. Cassady

Radiation Therapy Physics
Edited by A. R. Smith

Late Sequelae in Oncology
Edited by J. Dunst and R. Sauer

Mediastinal Tumors. Update 1995
Edited by D. E. Wood and C. R. Thomas, Jr.

**Thermoradiotherapy
and Thermochemotherapy**
Volume 1:
Biology, Physiology, and Physics
Volume 2:
Clinical Applications
Edited by M.H. Seegenschmiedt,
P. Fessenden, and C.C. Vernon

**Carcinoma of the Prostate
Innovations in Management**
Edited by Z. Petrovich, L. Baert,
and L.W. Brady

**Radiation Oncology
of Gynecological Cancers**
Edited by H.W. Vahrson

**Carcinoma of the Bladder
Innovations in Management**
Edited by Z. Petrovich, L. Baert,
and L.W. Brady

**Blood Perfusion and
Microenvironment of Human Tumors
Implications for Clinical Radiooncology**
Edited by M. Molls and P. Vaupel

**Radiation Therapy of Benign Diseases
A Clinical Guide**
2nd Revised Edition
S. E. Order and S. S. Donaldson

**Carcinoma of the Kidney and Testis,
and Rare Urologic Malignancies
Innovations in Management**
Edited by Z. Petrovich, L. Baert,
and L.W. Brady

**Progress and Perspectives in the
Treatment of Lung Cancer**
Edited by P. Van Houtte,
J. Klastersky, and P. Rocmans

**Combined Modality Therapy of
Central Nervous System Tumors**
Edited by Z. Petrovich, L. W. Brady,
M. L. Apuzzo, and M. Bamberg

**Age-Related Macular Degeneration
Current Treatment Concepts**
Edited by W. A. Alberti, G. Richard,
and R. H. Sagerman

**Radiotherapy of Intraocular
and Orbital Tumors**
2nd Revised Edition
Edited by R. H. Sagerman,
and W. E. Alberti

**Modification of Radiation Response
Cytokines, Growth Factors,
and Other Biolgical Targets**
Edited by C. Nieder, L. Milas,
and K. K. Ang

Radiation Oncology for Cure and Palliation
R. G. Parker, N. A. Janjan,
and M. T. Selch

**Clinical Target Volumes in Conformal and
Intensity Modulated Radiation Therapy
A Clinical Guide to Cancer Treatment**
Edited by V. Grégoire, P. Scalliet,
and K. K. Ang

**Advances in Radiation Oncology
in Lung Cancer**
Edited by Branislav Jeremić

New Technologies in Radiation Oncology
Edited by W. Schlegel, T. Bortfeld,
and A.-L. Grosu

Technical Basis of Radiation Therapy
4th Revised Edition
Edited by S. H. Levitt, J. A. Purdy, C. A.
Perez, and S. Vijayakumar

**Late Effects of Cancer Treatment on
Normal Tissues**
Edited by P. Rubin, L. S. Constine,
L. B. Marks, and P. Okunieff

**Clinical Practice of Radiation Therapy for
Benign Diseases Contemporary Concepts
and Clinical Results**
Edited by M. H. Seegenschmiedt,
H.-B. Makoski, K.-R. Trott, and
L. W. Brady

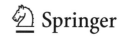

MEDICAL RADIOLOGY Diagnostic Imaging and Radiation Oncology
Titles in the series already published

DIAGNOSTIC IMAGING

Innovations in Diagnostic Imaging
Edited by J. H. Anderson

Radiology of the Upper Urinary Tract
Edited by E. K. Lang

The Thymus - Diagnostic Imaging, Functions, and Pathologic Anatomy
Edited by E. Walter, E. Willich, and W. R. Webb

Interventional Neuroradiology
Edited by A. Valavanis

Radiology of the Pancreas
Edited by A. L. Baert,
co-edited by G. Delorme

Radiology of the Lower Urinary Tract
Edited by E. K. Lang

Magnetic Resonance Angiography
Edited by I. P. Arlart, G. M. Bongartz, and G. Marchal

Contrast-Enhanced MRI of the Breast
S. Heywang-Köbrunner and R. Beck

Spiral CT of the Chest
Edited by M. Rémy-Jardin and J. Rémy

Radiological Diagnosis of Breast Diseases
Edited by M. Friedrich and E.A. Sickles

Radiology of the Trauma
Edited by M. Heller and A. Fink

Biliary Tract Radiology
Edited by P. Rossi,
co-edited by M. Brezi

Radiological Imaging of Sports Injuries
Edited by C. Masciocchi

Modern Imaging of the Alimentary Tube
Edited by A. R. Margulis

Diagnosis and Therapy of Spinal Tumors
Edited by P. R. Algra, J. Valk, and J. J. Heimans

Interventional Magnetic Resonance Imaging
Edited by J. F. Debatin and G. Adam

Abdominal and Pelvic MRI
Edited by A. Heuck and M. Reiser

Orthopedic Imaging
Techniques and Applications
Edited by A. M. Davies and H. Pettersson

Radiology of the Female Pelvic Organs
Edited by E. K.Lang

Magnetic Resonance of the Heart and Great Vessels
Clinical Applications
Edited by J. Bogaert, A.J. Duerinckx, and F. E. Rademakers

Modern Head and Neck Imaging
Edited by S. K. Mukherji and J. A. Castelijns

Radiological Imaging of Endocrine Diseases
Edited by J. N. Bruneton
in collaboration with B. Padovani and M.-Y. Mourou

Trends in Contrast Media
Edited by H. S. Thomsen,
R. N. Muller, and R. F. Mattrey

Functional MRI
Edited by C. T. W. Moonen and P. A. Bandettini

Radiology of the Pancreas
2nd Revised Edition
Edited by A. L. Baert. Co-edited by G. Delorme and L. Van Hoe

Emergency Pediatric Radiology
Edited by H. Carty

Spiral CT of the Abdomen
Edited by F. Terrier, M. Grossholz, and C. D. Becker

Liver Malignancies
Diagnostic and
Interventional Radiology
Edited by C. Bartolozzi and R. Lencioni

Medical Imaging of the Spleen
Edited by A. M. De Schepper and F. Vanhoenacker

Radiology of Peripheral Vascular Diseases
Edited by E. Zeitler

Diagnostic Nuclear Medicine
Edited by C. Schiepers

Radiology of Blunt Trauma of the Chest
P. Schnyder and M. Wintermark

Portal Hypertension
Diagnostic Imaging-Guided Therapy
Edited by P. Rossi
Co-edited by P. Ricci and L. Broglia

Recent Advances in Diagnostic Neuroradiology
Edited by Ph. Demaerel

Virtual Endoscopy and Related 3D Techniques
Edited by P. Rogalla, J. Terwisscha Van Scheltinga, and B. Hamm

Multislice CT
Edited by M. F. Reiser, M. Takahashi, M. Modic, and R. Bruening

Pediatric Uroradiology
Edited by R. Fotter

Transfontanellar Doppler Imaging in Neonates
A. Couture and C. Veyrac

Radiology of AIDS
A Practical Approach
Edited by J.W.A.J. Reeders and P.C. Goodman

CT of the Peritoneum
Armando Rossi and Giorgio Rossi

Magnetic Resonance Angiography
2nd Revised Edition
Edited by I. P. Arlart,
G. M. Bongratz, and G. Marchal

Pediatric Chest Imaging
Edited by Javier Lucaya and Janet L. Strife

Applications of Sonography in Head and Neck Pathology
Edited by J. N. Bruneton
in collaboration with C. Raffaelli and O. Dassonville

Imaging of the Larynx
Edited by R. Hermans

3D Image Processing
Techniques and Clinical Applications
Edited by D. Caramella and C. Bartolozzi

Imaging of Orbital and Visual Pathway Pathology
Edited by W. S. Müller-Forell

Pediatric ENT Radiology
Edited by S. J. King and A. E. Boothroyd

Radiological Imaging of the Small Intestine
Edited by N. C. Gourtsoyiannis

Imaging of the Knee
Techniques and Applications
Edited by A. M. Davies and V. N. Cassar-Pullicino

Perinatal Imaging
From Ultrasound to MR Imaging
Edited by Fred E. Avni

Radiological Imaging of the Neonatal Chest
Edited by V. Donoghue

Diagnostic and Interventional Radiology in Liver Transplantation
Edited by E. Bücheler, V. Nicolas, C. E. Broelsch, X. Rogiers, and G. Krupski

Radiology of Osteoporosis
Edited by S. Grampp

Imaging Pelvic Floor Disorders
Edited by C. I. Bartram and J. O. L. DeLancey
Associate Editors: S. Halligan, F. M. Kelvin, and J. Stoker

Imaging of the Pancreas
Cystic and Rare Tumors
Edited by C. Procacci and A. J. Megibow

High Resolution Sonography of the Peripheral Nervous System
Edited by S. Peer and G. Bodner

Imaging of the Foot and Ankle
Techniques and Applications
Edited by A. M. Davies, R. W. Whitehouse, and J. P. R. Jenkins

Radiology Imaging of the Ureter
Edited by F. Joffre, Ph. Otal, and M. Soulie

Imaging of the Shoulder
Techniques and Applications
Edited by A. M. Davies and J. Hodler

Radiology of the Petrous Bone
Edited by M. Lemmerling and S. S. Kollias

Interventional Radiology in Cancer
Edited by A. Adam, R. F. Dondelinger, and P. R. Mueller

Duplex and Color Doppler Imaging of the Venous System
Edited by G. H. Mostbeck

Multidetector-Row CT of the Thorax
Edited by U. J. Schoepf

Functional Imaging of the Chest
Edited by H.-U. Kauczor

Radiology of the Pharynx and the Esophagus
Edited by O. Ekberg

Radiological Imaging in Hematological Malignancies
Edited by A. Guermazi

Imaging and Intervention in Abdominal Trauma
Edited by R. F. Dondelinger

Multislice CT
2nd Revised Edition
Edited by M. F. Reiser, M. Takahashi, M. Modic, and C. R. Becker

Intracranial Vascular Malformations and Aneurysms
From Diagnostic Work-Up to Endovascular Therapy
Edited by M. Forsting

Radiology and Imaging of the Colon
Edited by A. H. Chapman

Coronary Radiology
Edited by M. Oudkerk

Dynamic Contrast-Enhanced Magnetic Resonance Imaging in Oncology
Edited by A. Jackson, D. L. Buckley, and G. J. M. Parker

Imaging in Treatment Planning for Sinonasal Diseases
Edited by R. Maroldi and P. Nicolai

Clinical Cardiac MRI
With Interactive CD-ROM
Edited by J. Bogaert, S. Dymarkowski, and A. M. Taylor

Focal Liver Lesions
Detection, Characterization, Ablation
Edited by R. Lencioni, D. Cioni, and C. Bartolozzi

Multidetector-Row CT Angiography
Edited by C. Catalano and R. Passariello

Paediatric Musculoskeletal Diseases
With an Emphasis on Ultrasound
Edited by D. Wilson

Contrast Media in Ultrasonography
Basic Principles and Clinical Applications
Edited by Emilio Quaia

MR Imaging in White Matter Diseases of the Brain and Spinal Cord
Edited by M. Filippi, N. De Stefano, V. Dousset, and J. C. McGowan

Diagnostic Nuclear Medicine
2nd Revised Edition
Edited by C. Schiepers

Imaging of the Kidney Cancer
Edited by A. Guermazi

Magnetic Resonance Imaging in Ischemic Stroke
Edited by R. von Kummer and T. Back

Imaging of the Hip & Bony Pelvis
Techniques and Applications
Edited by A. M. Davies, K. J. Johnson, and R. W. Whitehouse

Imaging of Occupational and Environmental Disorders of the Chest
Edited by P. A. Gevenois and P. De Vuyst

Contrast Media
Safety Issues and ESUR Guidelines
Edited by H. S. Thomsen

Virtual Colonoscopy
A Practical Guide
Edited by P. Lefere and S. Gryspeerdt

Vascular Embolotherapy
A Comprehensive Approach
Volume 1: *General Principles, Chest, Abdomen, and Great Vessels*
Edited by J. Golzarian. Co-edited by S. Sun and M. J. Sharafuddin

Vascular Embolotherapy
A Comprehensive Approach
Volume 2: *Oncology, Trauma, Gene Therapy, Vascular Malformations, and Neck*
Edited by J. Golzarian. Co-edited by S. Sun and M. J. Sharafuddin

Head and Neck Cancer Imaging
Edited by R. Hermans

Vascular Interventional Radiology
Current Evidence in Endovascular Surgery
Edited by M. G. Cowling

Ultrasound of the Gastrointestinal Tract
Edited by G. Maconi and G. Bianchi Porro

Imaging of Orthopedic Sports Injuries
Edited by F. M. Vanhoenacker, M. Maas, J. L. M. A. Gielen

Parallel Imaging in Clinical MR Applications
Edited by S. O. Schoenberg, O. Dietrich, and F. M. Reiser

MR and CT of the Female Pelvis
Edited by B. Hamm and R. Forstner

Ultrasound of the Musculoskeletal System
S. Bianchi and C. Martinoli

Spinal Imaging
Diagnostic Imaging of the Spine and Spinal Cord
Edited by J. W. M. Van Goethem, L. Van den Hauwe, and P. M. Parizel

Radiation Dose from Adult and Pediatric Multidetector Computed Tomography
Edited by D. Tack and P. A. Gevenois

Computed Tomography of the Lung
A Pattern Approach
J. A. Verschakelen and W. De Wever

Clinical Functional MRI
Presurgical Functional Neuroimaging
Edited bei C. Stippich

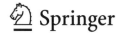

Printed by Publishers' Graphics LLC USA